The Simple Hypothyroidism Diet Cookbook

80 Plus Nutritious Recipes for Thyroid Disorder

Copyright © 2024 by Laura Thompson. All rights reserved.

The content, in this book is protected by copyright law. Any reproduction or distribution without written consent from the publisher is strictly prohibited.

The author and publisher have taken precautions to ensure the accuracy of the information provided; however, they do not accept responsibility for any errors or omissions that may occur.

It's important to note that the information shared in this book is for purposes and should not be considered as advice. Readers are encouraged to seek guidance from a healthcare expert before implementing any changes, to their diet or lifestyle.

ISBN: 9798339101833

Contents

Introduction 1

    How Common Is Hypothyroidism? 2

Overview of Hypothyrodism 5

    Signs and Symptoms of Hypothyroidism (Underactive Thyroid) 6

    Causes and Risk Factors of Hypothyroidism 20

    How Hypothyroidism Is Diagnosed 31

    How Hypothyroidism Is Treated 45

    Diet and Hypothyroidism 76

1   Hypothyroidism Recipes 98

    1.1   Berry Green Smoothie 98

    1.2   Mixed Berry Banana Smoothie 98

    1.3   Green Monster Smoothie 99

    1.4   Goji Grapefruit Parsley Smoothie 100

    1.5   Spinach Peach Smoothie 101

    1.6   Silky Choco-Hazelnut Smoothie 102

    1.7   Cashew Butter Green Smoothie 103

1.8   Super green Basil Smoothie 105

1.9   Pumpkin Smoothie 106

1.10 Turmeric Chai Latte (dairy free) 108

1.11 Overnight Chocolate Chia Seed Pudding 109

1.12 Green Plantain (Grain-Free) Pancake 111

1.13 Fruit & Coconut Yogurt Parfait 113

1.14 Coconut Flour Porridge 115

1.15 Banana Pancakes 116

1.16 Coconut Flour Pancakes With Blueberry Maple Syrup 117

1.17 Banana Breakfast Pancakes 119

1.18 Banana Muffins 120

1.19 Carrot Orange Muffins 122

1.20 Savory Oatmeal Sweet Potatoes 124

1.21 Quinoa Stir Fry 126

1.22 Almond Flour Zucchini Apple Pancakes 128

1.23 Sweet Potato Fritters 130

1.24 Sweet potato Hash {Greek Style} With Feta Cheese & Eggs 131

1.25 Coconut Macadamia Granola 133

1.26 Chocolate Cherry Almond Granola 136

1.27 Cranberry Zinger 138

1.28 Basted Eggs Over Sausage & Pepper Hash ...139

1.29 Mini Mushroom and Sausage Quiches 141

1.30 Lamb Hash with Carrot & Celery Root 143

1.31 Herbed Lamb Sausage 145

1.32 Eggnog – Dairy & Egg free 147

1.33 Simple Bone Broth 148

1.34 Ginger-Chicken Noodle Soup 150

1.35 Split Pea Soup with Smoked Ham 152

1.36 Tomato, Sausage & Fennel Soup 154

1.37 Orange Velvet Soup 156

1.38 Thai Chicken Soup with Coconut Milk 158

1.39 Pumpkin Soup 161

1.40 Yummy Kale Salad 162

1.41	Roasted Beet & Carrot Salad with Herbs	163
1.42	Roasted Radish & Seaweed Salad	166
1.43	Quick Sauerkraut Salad	168
1.44	Greek Yogurt Tuna Salad	169
1.45	Zucchini and Anchovy Quick Salad	170
1.46	Brown Rice Salad with Shrimp & Avocado	171
1.47	Lentil and Green Pea Salad	174
1.48	Chickpea & Bulgur Salad	176
1.49	Asian Bok Choy and Mushroom Salad	178
1.50	Middle Eastern Mason jar Salad	179
1.51	One Pot Cheesy Taco Skillet	181
1.52	Lamb Stew with Mushrooms & Red Wine	182
1.53	Lentil Stew	185
1.54	Vegetable Soup with Mediterranean Salad	187
1.55	Slow Cooker Vegetarian Chili	190
1.56	Pumpkin Turkey Chili	192
1.57	Sweet & Spicy Quinoa Chili	194

1.58 Easy Mexican Black Beans with Greens 196

1.59 Summer Squash Skillet...197

1.60 Baked Risotto Primavera...................................201

1.61 Rosemary Roasted Potatoes and Tomatoes ..203

1.62 Moroccan Bean..204

1.63 Saucy Vegan Vegetable & Chickpea Curry....206

1.64 Curried Lamb & Fennel Meatballs in Tomato Sauce 209

1.65 Moroccan Chicken 211

1.66 Quinoa Crusted Chicken Parmesan................213

1.67 Chicken Cilantro...215

1.68 Maple-Chili Glazed Pork Medallions...............218

1.69 Southwestern Steak and Peppers.....................220

1.70 Smoky Stuffed Peppers 222

1.71 Steamed Artichokes with Garlic Cashew Aioli 224

1.72 Sweet Italian Sausage 225

1.73 Loaded Lasagna 227

1.74 Stuffed Delicata Squash with Sausage, Greens, & Garlic 231

1.75 Healthy Chipotle Chicken Sweet Potato Skins 234

1.76 Loaded Chili 237

1.77 Baked Salmon 240

1.78 Salmon, Sweet Potato & Watercress Salad with Turmeric Cream 241

1.79 Sizzled Citrus Shrimp 243

1.80 Shrimp, Zucchini & Pesto Angel Hair Pasta . 245

1.81 Roasted Cod, Tomatoes, Orange, & Onions 246

1.82 Grilled Rosemary-Salmon Skewers 248

1.83 Arugula Lemon Pesto 250

Bonus chapter 252

Ways to Boost Your Energy with Hypothyroidism . 252

Weight Gain and Hypothyroidism 257

Conclusion 262

INTRODUCTION

Hypothyroidism occurs when the thyroid gland does not produce enough thyroid hormones. An underactive thyroid gland can lead to weight gain, tiredness, and feeling cold constantly.

Thyroid hormones (thyroxine) regulate metabolism, which is how the body uses energy. If thyroxine levels are low, many of the body's functions slow down.

About 4.6% of the population of the United States of America ages 12 years and above have hypothyroidism.

The thyroid gland is found in the front of the neck below the larynx, or voice box, and has two lobes, one on each side of the windpipe.

The production of thyroid hormones is regulated by thyroid-stimulating hormone (TSH), which is made by the pituitary gland.

This, in turn, is regulated by the hypothalamus, a region of the brain. TSH ensures that enough thyroid hormones are made to meet the needs of the body.

How Common Is Hypothyroidism?

Hypothyroidism is a common endocrine (hormonal) disorder. In the United States, 1 in 300 people have been diagnosed with hypothyroidism.

Rates of hypothyroidism have been increasing in recent years. Levothyroxine, the most commonly used treatment for hypothyroidism, is one of the most prescribed drugs in the United States.

More than 12% of the U.S. population will develop a thyroid condition at some point during their lifetime.

Hypothyroidism by Ethnicity

Studies on the incidence of hypothyroidism in different ethnicities is limited, however, it has been established that White people are more likely to be diagnosed with hypothyroidism than other ethnicities.

In one Brazilian study, nearly 17 out of 100 White women vs. nearly 7 out of 100 Black women were diagnosed with hypothyroidism.

Hypothyroidism by Age and Gender

Hypothyroidism is 8 to 9 times more likely to develop in women than men. The risk of developing hypothyroidism increases in people who are pregnant, have recently given birth, or are going through menopause.

As people age, the risk of developing hypothyroidism increases as well. Hypothyroidism is more prevalent in people over 60.

Overview of Hypothyrodism

Hypothyroidism or underactive thyroid is a condition that occurs when your thyroid gland does not make enough thyroid hormone. The thyroid gland is a butterfly-shaped organ located in the neck, which plays an important role in regulating your hormones, metabolism, and body temperature.

Having an underlying autoimmune disease, taking certain medications, and undergoing radiation are some causes of hypothyroidism. Historically, about 5% of people in the U.S. have received a diagnosis for an underactive thyroid. However, a 2023 study reported that the number of people with hypothyroidism is increasing and researchers estimate that 11.4% of people had this condition in 2019.

While there is no cure for hypothyroidism, the good news is that you can treat the condition with medications that can help you restore your hormone levels and thyroid function.

Signs and Symptoms of Hypothyroidism (Underactive Thyroid)

Hypothyroidism, or an underactive thyroid, is when the thyroid gland produces too few hormones. Low levels of thyroid hormones can cause a wide range of signs and symptoms, from changes in mental functioning to digestive issues.

The thyroid is a butterfly-shaped gland that sits in front of the neck. Thyroid hormones play a vital role in regulating metabolism and energy use and affect almost all of the body's organs.

In this section, we describe 12 common signs and symptoms of hypothyroidism. We also discuss the later symptoms of untreated hypothyroidism, how common hypothyroidism is, and when to see a doctor.

Fatigue

Fatigue is one of the most common symptoms of hypothyroidism.

Many people with the condition report feeling so exhausted that they are unable to go about their day as usual.

The fatigue occurs regardless of how much sleep a person gets or how many daytime naps they take. Treatment for hypothyroidism usually improves people's energy levels and functioning.

Weight gain

Thyroid hormones help to regulate body weight, food intake, and the metabolism of fat and sugar. People with low levels of thyroid hormones can experience weight gain and an increase in body mass index (BMI).

Even mild cases of hypothyroidism may increase the risk of weight gain and obesity. People with the condition often report having a puffy face as well as excess weight around the stomach or other areas of the body.

Sore muscles and joints

Hypothyroidism can affect a person's muscles and joints in numerous ways, causing:

- aches
- pains

- stiffness
- swelling of the joints
- tenderness
- weakness

Research also suggests a link between thyroid disorders and rheumatoid arthritis, which is an autoimmune condition that causes painful swelling in the lining of the joints. Effective treatment for both conditions will help people manage their symptoms.

Mood and memory changes

It is common for individuals with untreated hypothyroidism to experience:

- anxiety
- depression

- apathy, or general lack of interest or feelings of indifference
- impaired memory function
- less attentiveness and concentration
- low moods
- slower thinking and speech

These symptoms can occur because the brain requires thyroid hormones to function correctly. Research shows that low levels of thyroid hormones can cause changes in brain structure and functioning.

These brain changes can reverse once a person begins treatment.

Feeling cold

Hypothyroidism can slow down metabolism, leading to a drop in core body temperature. As such, some people with low levels of thyroid hormones may feel cold all the time or have a low tolerance to the cold.

This feeling of coldness can persist, even when in a warm room or during the summer months. People with hypothyroidism often report having cold hands or feet, although they may feel their whole body is cold.

These symptoms are not exclusive to hypothyroidism, however. Circulation problems or anemia can also cause people to feel chilly.

Constipation

Digestion is another body function that can slow down due to hypothyroidism.

Studies report that an underactive thyroid can cause problems with movement through the gut and the activity of the stomach, small intestine, and colon.

These digestive changes cause some people to experience constipation.

Doctors typically define constipation as having fewer than three bowel movements a week. A person may also have hard stools, difficulty passing stool, or a feeling of being unable to empty the rectum fully.

High cholesterol

Thyroid hormones play a vital role in removing excess cholesterol from the body via the liver. Low hormone levels mean that the liver struggles to carry out this function and blood cholesterol levels can increase.

Research suggests that up to 13 percent of individuals with high cholesterol also have an underactive thyroid. As a result, many experts recommend that doctors routinely test people with high cholesterol for hypothyroidism.

Treating the thyroid problem may help reduce cholesterol levels, even in those who do not take cholesterol-lowering drugs.

Slow heart rate

People with hypothyroidism may also have a slower heart rate, or bradycardia. Low thyroid levels can affect the heart in other ways too. These effects may include:

- changes in blood pressure
- variations in heart rhythm

- less elastic arteries

Bradycardia can cause weakness, dizziness, and breathing problems. Without treatment, this heart condition may result in serious complications, such as high or low blood pressure or heart failure.

Hair loss

Untreated hormone disorders, including thyroid problems, can contribute to hair loss. This is because thyroid hormones are essential for the growth and health of hair follicles. Hypothyroidism may cause hair loss from the:

- scalp
- eyebrows
- legs

- other body parts

People with thyroid problems are also more prone to developing alopecia, which is an autoimmune condition that causes hair to fall out in patches.

Dry skin and weak hair and nails

An underactive thyroid affects the skin in various ways and can cause symptoms, such as:

- dry, coarse skin
- paleness
- thin, scaly skin

People with hypothyroidism may also develop dry, brittle, and coarse hair or dull, thin nails that break easily.

These symptoms usually clear up once people begin thyroid hormone therapy.

Goiter

A goiter is an enlargement of the thyroid gland that appears as a swelling at the base of the neck. Other goiter symptoms include:

- **a cough**
- **hoarseness**
- **problems swallowing and breathing**

Many thyroid problems can result in a goiter, including Hashimoto's thyroiditis, which is an autoimmune condition that damages the thyroid gland, stopping it producing enough hormones.

Other causes include underactive thyroid and, less commonly in the United States, iodine deficiency.

Menstrual changes

People with an underactive thyroid may experience heavy or irregular menstrual periods or spotting between periods.

According to the Society of Menstrual Cycle Research, hypothyroidism causes these problems because it affects other hormones that play a role in menstruation, such as by:

- impairing the degradation of estrogen
- reducing the amount of sex hormone-binding globulin

Late symptoms

Hypothyroidism develops slowly and symptoms may go unnoticed for a long time. In the event that hypothyroidism is left untreated, a person may develop the following late symptoms:

- decreased taste and smell
- hoarseness
- puffy face, hands, and feet
- slow speech
- thickening of the skin
- thinning of eyebrows
- low body temperature
- slow heart rate

How common is it?

According to the National Institute of Diabetes and Digestive and Kidney Diseases, hypothyroidism affects around 4.6 percent of people aged 12 years or older in the U.S. However, most of these individuals experience only mild symptoms.

Hypothyroidism is more likely to occur in women and people over 60 years of age.

Other risk factors include:

- a personal or family history of thyroid problems
- previous thyroid surgery or radiation treatment to the neck or chest
- having been pregnant recently

other health conditions, such as Turner syndrome, Sjögren's syndrome, or certain autoimmune conditions

Causes and Risk Factors of Hypothyroidism

Hypothyroidism may develop for a number of different reasons, the most common being an autoimmune attack on the thyroid gland, called Hashimoto's thyroiditis. Hypothyroidism may also be the result of taking a medication like lithium, genetics, or an underlying pituitary gland problem.

Understanding the "why" behind a diagnosis of hypothyroidism is critical to moving forward with a proper treatment plan. While some people may require lifelong thyroid hormone replacement, others may have a short-lived case of hypothyroidism (for example, postpartum thyroiditis), need to stop taking a medication, or require further diagnostic tests like imaging of the pituitary gland.

Common Causes

Hashimoto's thyroiditis is the leading cause of hypothyroidism in the United States.

In Hashimoto's, antibodies react against proteins in your thyroid gland, causing gradual destruction of the gland itself, rendering it unable to produce the thyroid hormones your body needs.

Hashimoto's thyroiditis is more common in women, and while it may occur at any age, it's more common as people get older. For women, Hashimoto's often develops during pregnancy, after delivery, or around the time of menopause.

Other causes of hypothyroidism include:

Surgery

People with hyperthyroidism, thyroid nodules, or thyroid cancer may need to have surgery. If all of the thyroid gland is surgically removed, a person will be hypothyroid and require lifelong thyroid hormone replacement medications. If only part of the thyroid gland is removed, there is a good chance that it will still be able to make sufficient thyroid hormone.

Radiation

Instead of thyroid surgery or antithyroid medication, some people with hyperthyroidism are treated with radioactive iodine, which will destroy the thyroid gland, rendering a person hypothyroid. People who undergo radiation treatment for Hodgkin's lymphoma or head and neck cancer are also at risk of developing hypothyroidism.

Thyroiditis

Thyroiditis describes thyroid gland inflammation and is a general term for a variety of thyroid conditions.

Hashimoto's disease is the most common type of thyroiditis and is caused by an autoimmune attack.

Another example of thyroiditis is subacute thyroiditis (also called de Quervain's thyroiditis), which is believed to be caused by a virus. With this type of thyroiditis, a person experiences hyperthyroidism followed by hypothyroidism, in addition to a tender thyroid gland.

Certain Drugs

Certain medications may trigger hypothyroidism. These medications include:

- Lithium
- Amiodarone
- Thionamides (antithyroid drugs)
- Interferon-alpha
- Interleukin-2

Certain cancer drugs (tyrosine kinase inhibitors and checkpoint inhibitor immunotherapies)

Iodine Excess or Deficiency

Too much iodine (for example, from dietary supplements that contain kelp) can cause or worsen hypothyroidism. In addition, a deficiency of iodine, which is seen in some people in underdeveloped countries, may cause hypothyroidism. Iodine is necessary for the production of thyroid hormone and is found in foods, like dairy products, chicken, beef, pork, fish, and iodized salt.

Congenital Hypothyroidism

Some babies are born without a thyroid gland or with only a partial thyroid gland. Since there is no thyroid gland (or not enough) to produce thyroid hormone, hypothyroidism develops, which is serious and requires treatment with a thyroid hormone pill.

Pituitary Gland Problem

The pituitary gland is located in the brain and stimulates other glands within the body, like the thyroid gland, to release hormones. If the pituitary gland is damaged by a brain tumor, radiation, or brain surgery, it may not function well enough to signal the thyroid gland. This can then result in it becoming underactive. This type of hypothyroidism is called central or secondary hypothyroidism.

Infiltrative Diseases

Rarely, certain diseases, like hemochromatosis, can deposit abnormal substances (iron, in the case of hemochromatosis) in your pituitary gland, causing central hypothyroidism, or less commonly, your thyroid gland, causing primary hypothyroidism.

Besides hemochromatosis, sarcoidosis can cause granuloma deposition in the thyroid gland. There is also a rare condition called fibrous thyroiditis (or Riedel's thyroiditis), in which fibrotic tissue replaces normal thyroid tissue.

Genetics

Your DNA plays a role when it comes to developing autoimmune hypothyroidism, and this has been supported by a number of studies.

One German study found a 32-fold increased risk for developing Hashimoto's thyroiditis in children and a 21-fold increased risk in siblings of people with Hashimoto's thyroiditis.

When looking at the specific genes linked to Hashimoto's, scientists have found mutations in the genes for human leukocyte antigen (HLA), T-cell receptors, and other molecules involved in the immune system.

To further support the role of genes in developing Hashimoto's thyroiditis, people with Turner syndrome and Down syndrome (both of which are genetic in origin) have a higher than expected rate of autoimmune thyroid disease, especially Hashimoto's thyroiditis.

All said, though, it's important to remember that your genes are but one factor that help predict your risk of developing hypothyroidism. There are many other factors that come into play, like pregnancy or taking certain medications.

In the end, it's the combination of genes and an environmental trigger that predict a person's unique risk for developing hypothyroidism.

Risk Factors

Factors that increase a person's risk of developing hypothyroidism include:

- Being female
- Being of an older age
- Being Caucasian or Asian
- Having a family history of Hashimoto's thyroiditis or another autoimmune disease
- Having a personal history of an autoimmune disease (for example, adrenal insufficiency, rheumatoid arthritis, or type 1 diabetes)
- Being pregnant or postpartum

- Too much or too little iodine consumption
- Treated with radioactive iodine
- Received radiation to the neck or upper chest
- Underwent thyroid surgery
- Treated with certain medications (for example, lithium for bipolar disorder)

Evolving Risk Factors

Interestingly, research suggests that selenium deficiency may be linked to developing Hashimoto's thyroiditis and hypothyroidism. Moreover, having underlying headache disorders, like migraines, has been found to be associated with an increased risk of hypothyroidism, especially in obese women.

It's still unclear precisely how smoking affects the thyroid gland, although it's likely complex. While some studies suggest that cigarette smoking increases the risk of hypothyroidism in people with Hashimoto's thyroiditis, other research suggests that smoking is actually linked to a lower prevalence of hypothyroidism and a higher prevalence of hyperthyroidism.

How Hypothyroidism Is Diagnosed

If you have signs or symptoms of an underactive thyroid gland (called hypothyroidism), it's important to see your healthcare provider for a complete evaluation. In order to check for a thyroid problem, your practitioner will ask you questions about your personal and family medical history, perform a physical examination, and run blood tests (most notably, a thyroid-stimulating hormone, or TSH test).

If your medical professional diagnoses you with hypothyroidism, he will also want to know the cause of your thyroid dysfunction, as this will dictate your treatment plan. To unveil the "why" behind your hypothyroid diagnosis, you may need to undergo further testing, like an antibody blood test.

History and Examination

When you see a healthcare provider for the first time with signs or symptoms suspicious for hypothyroidism, you can expect to undergo a complete medical history and physical examination.

After reviewing any new symptoms that signal your body's metabolism may be slowing down (for example, drier skin, tiring more easily, cold intolerance, or constipation), your healthcare provider will ask specific questions about your medical history.

Questions Your Healthcare Provider May Ask

- Do you have another autoimmune disease, such as rheumatoid arthritis or type 1 diabetes?
- Do you have any family members who have hypothyroidism?
- Have you ever had thyroid surgery?
- Are you taking any medications that cause hypothyroidism like amiodarone or lithium?
- Are you taking any iodine-containing supplements?
- Have you ever had radiation to your neck to treat lymphoma or head and neck cancer?

In addition to taking a medical history, your healthcare provider will examine your thyroid for enlargement (called a goiter) and lumps (nodules). Your practitioner will also check for signs of hypothyroidism like a low blood pressure, low pulse, dry skin, swelling, and sluggish reflexes.

Labs and Tests

The diagnosis of hypothyroidism relies heavily on blood tests.

Thyroid-Stimulating Hormone (TSH)

The TSH test is the primary test used for the diagnosis and management of hypothyroidism.But different labs often have slightly different values for what is known as the "TSH reference range."

At many labs, the TSH reference range runs from 0.5 to 4.5. A TSH value of less than 0.5 is considered hyperthyroid, while a TSH value of more than 4.5 is considered potentially hypothyroid.

Different labs might use a lower limit of anywhere from 0.35 to 0.6, and an upper threshold of anywhere from 4.0 to 6.0.

In any case, it is important for you to be aware of the reference range at the lab where your blood is sent, so you know the standards by which you are being diagnosed.

If the initial TSH blood test is elevated, it's often repeated, and a free thyroxine T4 test is also drawn.

Free Thyroxine (T4)

If the TSH is high and the free T4 is low, a diagnosis of primary hypothyroidism is made.

If the TSH is high, but the free T4 is normal, a diagnosis of subclinical hypothyroidism is made. Treatment of subclinical hypothyroidism depends on a number of factors.

For example, your healthcare provider may treat your subclinical hypothyroidism if you have symptoms like fatigue, constipation, or depression, or you have another autoimmune disease, for example, celiac disease.

Age will also play a role in your healthcare provider's decision. Typically, there is a higher threshold for initiating thyroid hormone replacement medication in older adults; this is because their baseline TSH is at the upper limits of normal.

The presence of TPO antibodies (see below) also plays a role in your healthcare provider's decision. If you have subclinical hypothyroidism and positive TPO antibodies, your practitioner will likely initiate thyroid hormone treatment to prevent the progression of subclinical hypothyroidism into overt hypothyroidism.

The rare diagnosis of central or secondary hypothyroidism is a bit trickier. Central hypothyroidism suggests a pituitary gland or hypothalamus problem. These brain structures control the thyroid gland and may be damaged from tumors, infections, radiation, and infiltrative diseases like sarcoidosis, among other causes.

In central hypothyroidism, the TSH is low or normal and the free T4 is generally low-normal or low.

TPO Antibodies

Positive thyroid peroxidase (TPO) antibodies suggest a diagnosis of Hashimoto's thyroiditis, which is the most common cause of hypothyroidism in the United States.

These antibodies slowly attack the thyroid gland, so the development of hypothyroidism tends to be a gradual process, as the thyroid becomes less and less able to produce thyroid hormone.

This means that a person can have positive TPO antibodies, but a normal thyroid function for some time; in fact, it can take years for a person's thyroid function to decline to the point of being hypothyroid. Some people even have positive TPO antibodies and never progress to being hypothyroid.

While your healthcare provider will not likely treat you with thyroid hormone replacement medication if your TPO antibodies are positive but your TSH is within the normal reference range, he will likely monitor your TSH over time to make sure that's still appropriate.

Imaging

While blood tests are the primary means of diagnosing hypothyroidism, your healthcare provider may order a thyroid ultrasound if he notes (or simply wants to check for) a goiter or nodules on your physical examination. An ultrasound can help a practitioner determine the size of a nodule and whether it has features suspicious for cancer.

Sometimes, a needle biopsy (called a fine needle aspiration, or FNA) is performed to obtain a sample of the cells within a nodule. These cells can then be examined more closely under a microscope.

In the case of central hypothyroidism, imaging is done to examine the brain and pituitary gland. For instance, an MRI of the pituitary gland may reveal a tumor, like a pituitary adenoma.

Differential Diagnosis

The symptoms of hypothyroidism are highly variable and may be easily missed or mistaken for another medical condition.

Based on Symptoms

Depending on your unique symptoms, your healthcare provider will evaluate you for alternative medical conditions (especially if your TSH is normal). These may include:

- Anemia
- A viral infection (for example, mononucleosis or Lyme disease)
- Vitamin D deficiency
- Fibromyalgia
- Depression or anxiety
- Sleep apnea

- Liver or kidney disease
- Another autoimmune disease (for example celiac disease or rheumatoid arthritis)

Based on Blood Test Results

While primary hypothyroidism is the most likely culprit behind an elevated TSH, there are some other diagnoses your healthcare provider will keep in mind. For instance, thyroid blood tests that support a diagnosis of central hypothyroidism may actually be due to a nonthyroidal illness.

Nonthyroidal Illness

People who are hospitalized with a serious illness or who have undergone a bone marrow transplantation, major surgery, or heart attack may have thyroid function blood tests consistent with central hypothyroidism (a low TSH and low T4), yet their "nonthyroidal illness" does not generally warrant treatment.

Blood tests called reverse T3, a metabolite of T4, can be helpful in distinguishing between true central hypothyroidism and nonthyroidal illness. A reverse T3 is elevated in nonthyroidal illness.

In nonthyroidal illness, thyroid function blood tests should normalize once a person recovers from their illness. Although, some people develop an elevated TSH after recovery. In these people, repeating a TSH in four to six weeks usually reveals a normal TSH.

Untreated Adrenal Insufficiency

Hypothyroidism and adrenal insufficiency may coexist, as they do in a rare condition called autoimmune polyglandular syndrome. This syndrome results from autoimmune processes involving multiple glands, especially the thyroid gland (causing hypothyroidism) and adrenal glands (causing adrenal insufficiency).

One of the biggest dangers associated with this syndrome is treating the hypothyroidism (giving thyroid hormone replacement) before treating the hypoadrenalism (which requires corticosteroid treatment), as this can result in a life-threatening adrenal crisis.

Unfortunately, with this syndrome, the hypoadrenalism may be missed because of an elevated TSH and vague symptoms that overlap with those seen in hypothyroidism.

TSH-producing Pituitary Adenoma

If the TSH is elevated, it's essential that a free T4 is also checked. In primary hypothyroidism, the free T4 should be low, but if a person has a TSH-secreting pituitary tumor, the free T4 will be elevated.

Next Steps

Many people are diagnosed with hypothyroidism by their family healthcare provider or internist. However, primary care practitioners have varying experience in managing thyroid disease.

Your first task is to learn whether or not your primary care healthcare provider feels comfortable treating you, or if you should consult with an endocrinologist (a practitioner who specializes in treating hormone disorders).

In the end, you may see an endocrinologist once, and then have your primary care healthcare provider manage your thyroid disease moving forward. Alternatively, your endocrinologist may do all of your thyroid care year after year if this is the case.

How Hypothyroidism Is Treated

Thyroid hormone replacement with a prescription thyroid drug is the standard treatment for hypothyroidism (low thyroid hormones) caused by an underactive thyroid gland, surgically removed gland, or congenitally damaged or missing gland. Autoimmune Hashimoto's disease is the most common cause of hypothyroidism.

The goals of treatment include:

- Normalizing thyroid hormone levels, specifically, thyroxine (T4) and thyroid-stimulating hormone (TSH) levels

- Eliminating symptoms of hypothyroidism, like constipation, fatigue, and cold intolerance
- Halting and reversing any effects that hypothyroidism may be having on various organ systems (for example, elevated cholesterol levels)
- Reducing the size of a goiter, if present, as is sometimes the case with Hashimoto's disease

Levothyroxine (T4)

Hypothyroidism is treated with prescription oral thyroid hormone preparation (usually levothyroxine, a T4 preparation). The ideal dosage is sufficient enough to restore normal thyroid hormone levels without producing toxicity from too much thyroid hormone.

Formulations

There are different formulations of T4 made by different manufacturers. While all FDA-approved formulations are judged to be suitable, most experts recommend sticking to the same formulation, since the dosage equivalents may vary somewhat among different preparations.

In the United States, levothyroxine is available as generic levothyroxine, as well as Synthroid, Levothroid, and Levoxyl brand name tablets. Tirosint is a liquid gel cap form of levothyroxine that has been on the market since 2011.

Dosing

For young, healthy people, healthcare providers will generally begin with what is estimated to be a "full replacement dose" of T4 (that is, a dose that is supposed to completely restore thyroid function to normal). The full replacement dose is estimated according to body weight and, for most people, is between 50 and 200 micrograms (mcg) per day.

For older people or people who have coronary artery disease, thyroid replacement therapy is usually started gradually, beginning with 25 to 50 mcg daily and increasing over time.

T4 for Younger People

- Begin with a dose between 50 and 200 micrograms (mcg) per day
- Begins with a full replacement dose

T4 for Older People

- Begin with a dose between 25 and 50 micrograms (mcg) per day
- Dose begins low and gradually gets increased

Administration

You should take T4 on an empty stomach to prevent the absorption of the medication from being erratic. Healthcare providers usually recommend taking the medication first thing in the morning, then waiting at least an hour to eat breakfast or drink coffee. Taking the medication at bedtime, several hours after the last meal, also appears to work and can be a more convenient approach for some people.

Monitoring

TSH levels are monitored to help optimize the dose of T4. TSH stimulates the thyroid gland to make thyroid hormones. It is produced by the pituitary gland, and the body often adjusts the level of TSH in response to thyroid hormone levels.

So when thyroid hormone levels are low (as in hypothyroidism), the pituitary gland responds by increasing TSH levels. When hypothyroidism is adequately treated, TSH levels typically drop back down into the normal range. So, a mainstay in determining the best dose of T4 is measuring TSH levels.

How the Thyroid Gland Works

While symptoms of hypothyroidism usually begin to resolve within two weeks of initiating treatment, it takes about six weeks for TSH levels to stabilize. That is why

TSH levels are generally measured six weeks after treatment has begun.

If TSH levels remain above the target range, the dose of T4 is increased by about 12 to 25 mcg per day, and TSH levels are tested again after six more weeks. This process is continued until the TSH level reaches the desired range and symptoms are resolved.

Once the optimal dose of T4 is settled upon, TSH levels are measured every year or so thereafter, to make sure the treatment remains optimized.

Liothyronine (T3)

While the standard approach to treating hypothyroidism (T4 replacement) works for most people, some people continue to experience symptoms.

According to a 2016 study published in the Journal of Clinical Endocrinology and Metabolism, about 15% of people in the United States with hypothyroidism continue to have symptoms despite being treated for the disease.

Some practitioners may consider liothyronine (T3) as an add-on treatment for select individuals, though this is a matter of debate.

The Controversy

T4 is the major circulating thyroid hormone, but it is not the active form of the hormone. T4 is converted to T3 in the tissues as needed. And T3 is the thyroid hormone that does all the work. T4 is merely a prohormone a repository of potential T3 and a way of making sure that enough T3 can be created on a minute-to-minute basis as needed.

When you take T4 and not T3, the effects rely on your tissues to convert just the right amount of T4 to T3 at just the right place and at just the right time.

There is emerging evidence suggesting that some people with hypothyroidism might not have an efficient conversion of T4 to T3.11 When this is the case, despite the fact that T4 levels may be normal, T3 levels may be low, especially in the tissues, where T3 actually does its work.

Why T4 to T3 conversion may be abnormal in some people is, at this point, largely speculation although at least one group of patients has been identified with a genetic variant (in the diodinase 2 gene) that reduces the conversion of T4 to T3.

It appears that healthcare providers should be treating at least some people (albeit, a small group, most likely) who have hypothyroidism with both T4 and T3.

Formulations

Liothyronine is a synthetic form of T3, and it is available in a manufactured form as the brand Cytomel, and also as generic liothyronine.12 T3 can also be compounded.

Dosing

Calculation of appropriate doses of T3 is trickier than appropriately dosing T4. T4 is inactive, so if you take too much there is no immediate direct tissue effect. T3 is a different story, though, as it is the active thyroid hormone. So if you take too much T3, you can experience hyperthyroid effects directly a risk, for instance, to people with cardiac disease.

When adding T3 to T4 during thyroid replacement therapy, most experts recommend administering a ratio of T4:T3 between 13:1 to 16:1, which is the natural ratio of people without thyroid disease.

Monitoring

If you're taking combined T4/T3 therapy, your practitioner will usually check a TSH level six weeks after you begin treatment.5 T3 levels are not generally checked because currently available T3 formulations lead to wide fluctuations in T3 blood levels throughout the day.

Medications Used to Treat Thyroid Disease

Desiccated Thyroid Extract

Desiccated thyroid extract contains both thyroxine (T4) and triiododothyronine (T3), and is derived from the thyroid glands of pigs.

Formulations

Several brands of desiccated thyroid are available by prescription in the United States and in some other countries, including Nature thyroid, WP Thyroid, Armour Thyroid, a generic NP Thyroid (made by manufacturer Acella), and a Canadian natural thyroid from manufacturer Erfa.

Important Note

While desiccated thyroid extract is available as a prescription, it's rarely recommended by healthcare providers anymore, as there is no scientific evidence it has any benefits over synthetic T4.

Moreover, the ratio of T4 and T3 in desiccated thyroid extract (about 4 to 1) is not the same as the human ratio (about fourteen to 1). So, even though desiccated thyroid extract is often considered to be "natural," its ratio of T4-to-T3 hormone does not mimic that of human physiology.

For Infants

In an infant diagnosed with congenital hypothyroidism, the goals of treatment are to restore thyroid levels to normal as quickly and safely as possible. The quicker the thyroid levels are normalized, the better the cognitive and motor skills development of the infant.

Levothyroxine is the treatment of choice for congenital hypothyroidism.

Administration

Often, a liquid form of levothyroxine is given to infants. It's important to not mix the levothyroxine with soy infant formula or any calcium or iron-fortified preparations. Soy, calcium, and iron can all reduce the infant's ability to absorb the medication properly.

If levothyroxine tablets are given to an infant, parents should crush the levothyroxine tablet and mix it with breast milk, formula, or water that's fed to the baby.

Monitoring

Children being treated for congenital hypothyroidism are evaluated on a regular schedule, often every several months for at least the first three years of life.

According to the European Society for Paediatric Endocrinology, in congenital hypothyroidism, serum T4 or free T4 and TSH blood tests should be performed at the following times:

- Every one to three months during the first 12 months of life
- Every one to four months between 1 and 3 years of age
- Every six to 12 months thereafter until growth is complete
- Every two weeks after the initiation of T4 treatment, and every two weeks until TSH level is normalized
- Four to six weeks after any change in dose

At more frequent intervals when there's any concern about medication dosing or if there are any abnormal results

Permanent or lifelong congenital hypothyroidism can be established by imaging and ultrasound studies showing that the thyroid is missing or ectopic, or a defect in the ability to synthesize and/or secrete thyroid hormone is confirmed.

If permanent hypothyroidism has not been established, levothyroxine treatment may be discontinued for a month at age 3, and the child retested. If levels remain normal, transient hypothyroidism is the presumed diagnosis. If levels become abnormal, permanent hypothyroidism is diagnosed.

Children with transient congenital hypothyroidism who are taken off medication should have periodic thyroid evaluation and retesting, as these children face an increased risk of developing a thyroid problem throughout their lives.

During Pregnancy

Having sufficient thyroid hormone throughout pregnancy is necessary in order to protect your pregnancy and the health of your baby. The drug of choice during pregnancy is T4 since T3 does not cross the placenta and T4 is very important for fetal brain development.

Before Pregnancy

According to guidelines from American Thyroid Association, the dosage of thyroid hormone (levothyroxine) replacement medication for a woman with pre-existing hypothyroidism should be adjusted to aim for a TSH level below 2.5 mIU/L prior to conception.

During Pregnancy

The traditional reference range used by the healthcare provider to diagnose and manage hypothyroidism is significantly narrower in pregnancy.

The TSH level should be maintained at the following trimester-specific levels:

- First trimester: Between 0.1 and 2.5 mIU/L
- Second trimester: Between 0.2 to 3.0 mIU/L
- Third trimester: Between 0.3 to 3.0 mIU/L
- Managing Thyroid Problems During Pregnancy

Complementary Alternative Medicine (CAM)

In addition to the traditional treatment of your hypothyroidism with thyroid hormone replacement, implementing lifestyle habits, mind-body practices, and dietary changes in your health care can offer many benefits.

For example, some experts suggest that certain yoga poses (specifically, shoulder stands and inverted poses where the feet are elevated) may be beneficial to blood flow to the thyroid gland, or to the reduction of general stress that contributes to worsening symptoms of hypothyroidism.

Moreover, some people find that guided meditation is helpful for the thyroid, as are other stress-reducing strategies like prayer, gentle yoga, tai chi, and needlework.

Self-Treatment

It's important to note that self-treating your thyroid problem with supplements is not a good idea. Treating an underactive thyroid is a complex process that requires careful symptom and dose monitoring by a practitioner.

Keep in mind, as well, that supplements are not regulated by the government, and there is no scientific consensus that they are safe and effective. In other words, just because a supplement is "natural" or available without a prescription does not necessarily mean that it's harmless.

It's important to be open and honest with your healthcare provider from the start about your use of complementary therapies, so you can ensure that nothing you're doing (or want to try) will interfere with your thyroid care.

While some holistic or CAM practitioners may be able to recommend approaches to support your thyroid, immune and hormonal systems, it's important to be cautious of any product that's marketed as a "cure" for your disease, or marketed as being without side effects.

Goals of Natural Treatment

Natural treatments cannot cure hypothyroidism; instead, they are aimed at:

- Controlling inflammation and autoimmune triggers associated with autoimmune diseases
- Increasing hormone production

Natural Treatment Options

Natural treatments address lifestyle and environmental factors that may impact thyroid hormone production and symptoms. These treatments should be as individual as your type of hypothyroidism and symptoms are.

Natural Treatment Warning

Be aware that there may be risks involved in natural treatments like supplements and herbal remedies, and it's vital to speak to your healthcare provider before starting them.

Diet

Hypothyroidism symptoms like fatigue, weight gain, and bloating can be helped by eating a nutritious, balanced diet that supports a healthy weight.

Weight gain might not be avoided even when taking hypothyroid medications, but a calorie-balanced diet can help. A registered dietitian can help you come up with a healthy eating plan.

Additionally, there is a component of some foods called goitrogens that can affect thyroid health when eaten in high amounts. Goitrogens can inhibit the process by which iodine is incorporated into the thyroid hormones thyroxine (T4) and triiodothyronine (T3). Typically, this is the case only in people with iodine deficiency, which is rare in the United States.

These foods include the following, among others:

- Broccoli
- Cauliflower
- Kale
- Cabbage

- Soy products

Supplements

Some supplements support common deficiencies in people with hypothyroidism. The need for these depends on your levels of vitamins and minerals. Some potentially beneficial supplements include:

Vitamin B-12: Autoimmune thyroid disease is associated with autoimmune disorders, pernicious anemia, and atrophic gastritis, which can cause malabsorption of vitamin B-12. A lack of B-12 can cause symptoms like fatigue.

Zinc: Some research shows that zinc supplementation can affect thyroid function. More research is needed.

Selenium: In combination with zinc, selenium may have some effect on thyroid function. Selenium facilitates the conversion of T4 to the active T3.

Iodine: Thyroid hormones require iodine for production, but it must be obtained through diet or supplements. Most Americans get enough iodine through their diet, including in iodized salt.

Desiccated pig or cow thyroid should be avoided. Dried animal thyroid is sold as a supplement but can be dangerous, undertreating or overtreating your condition and making you susceptible to bovine spongiform encephalopathy (BSE or mad cow disease).

Iodine Poisoning

While iodine poisoning is rare, overconsuming iodine can be as equally problematic as not consuming enough.

Herbal Remedies

Herbs cannot heal a thyroid deficiency, and some can cause harm, so always speak to your healthcare provider before taking any.

Some herbal supplements work with the hormones in your body to bolster thyroid function, but if and how they work depends on your unique thyroid condition.

One such herb that may help is ashwagandha, a nightshade plant commonly used in Ayurveda practice. It has been shown to reduce thyroid hormone abnormalities in subclinical hypothyroidism in a few small human studies when taken at 600 mg per day.

Ashwagandha Warning

It is vital to be aware that ashwagandha can produce thyrotoxicosis, a severe form of hyperthyroidism.

Essential Oils

Essential oils have been studied for their use in people with hypothyroidism.

Fatigue is a common symptom of thyroid hormone deficiency, and essential oils when used for aromatherapy have been found to reduce feelings of fatigue.

Beyond its use in aromatherapy, essential oils do not have enough medical research supporting them in treating hypothyroidism. However, spearmint and peppermint oils may help with the symptoms of:

- Joint pain
- Nausea
- Indigestion

Acupuncture

Not many studies have been done on the use of acupuncture for hypothyroidism.

A 2018 review of the current research showed some promise for acupuncture to increase thyroid hormones in people with hypothyroidism. Additional benefits include:

- Reduction of sensitivity to pain and stress
- A calming effect
- Improving muscle stiffness and joint stability
- Increasing circulation

Reducing inflammation

Make sure to tell your acupuncturist that you have a thyroid condition before receiving treatment. Similarly, tell your healthcare provider about your acupuncture treatments.

Meditation and Yoga

Some experts suggest that specific yoga poses 1increase blood flow to the thyroid gland, such as shoulder stands and inverted poses where the feet are elevated above the heart. Yoga is also thought to reduce the stress that can make the symptoms of hypothyroidism worse.

Similarly, guided meditation might be helpful for the thyroid as a stress reducer.

Combined Treatment Approach

If you are considering taking any natural treatment whether it be an herb, dietary supplement, essential oil, or acupuncture it's important to talk to your healthcare provider, who can help you weigh the potential risks and benefits for your unique case.

Often, gentle and safe options such as yoga and vitamin or mineral supplements are beneficial when combined with conventional medications and treatments prescribed by your healthcare provider.

In general, follow a healthy eating plan with:

- Plenty of fruits and vegetables
- Lean protein
- Complex carbohydrates

- Aim to get sufficient sleep and exercise as well.

Naturopathic Healthcare Providers

If your healthcare provider is unfamiliar with supplements or herbal therapies that interest you, you can seek the advice of a naturopathic healthcare provider. Just be sure the healthcare provider treating your thyroid disease is kept up to date about these treatments.

Diet and Hypothyroidism

When you are living with hypothyroidism (an underactive thyroid), figuring out what to eat can be a confusing process. This is especially true if you are trying to lose weight or battling symptoms of hypothyroidism, like bloating or fatigue.

The foods you eat can play an important role in managing the disease.

This section offers tips to improve your diet and help ease hypothyroidism symptoms.

Protecting Thyroid Function

Goitrogens are substances found in foods that may interfere with thyroid hormone production, especially for people with iodine deficiency, which is rare in the United States.

Goitrogen-containing foods, like broccoli, cauliflower, and cabbage, release a compound called goitrin when they are hydrolyzed (broken down chemically). However, when heated, this compound is typically eliminated. Talk with a healthcare provider about the specific servings of goitrogenic foods that are best for you.

What About Soy?

Soy is possibly goitrogenic food in the setting of iodine deficiency.

If you have iodine deficiency and consume large quantities of soy products, your thyroid may be affected. However, studies have shown soy is not a goitrogen if you have enough iodine in your body.

Changing Your Eating Habits

There is no one-size-fits-all approach to eating, but strict calorie counting or macronutrient counting is usually not recommended. This can often lead to disordered eating and an inability to understand hunger cues. In addition, drastic weight loss can result in muscle loss and a slower metabolism.

Making small, sustainable changes can help you stick to a new way of eating for good. When you consume nutrient-dense foods, such as vegetables, whole grains, lean proteins, and healthy fats, you will feel satisfied without depriving yourself.

Break Down Your Plate

Focus on your plate, and include fat, fiber, and protein at each meal. Fill 50% of your plate with non-starchy vegetables, 25% with lean protein, and 25% with starches from foods such as whole grains or legumes, which include nuts, beans, and seeds.

Choose Fiber-Rich Foods

A meal plan rich in fiber is associated with a reduced risk of constipation (which commonly affects people with hypothyroidism), heart disease, diabetes, and certain types of cancer while improving weight loss.

Fiber is found in plants, such as fruits, vegetables, nuts, seeds, and whole grains.

Drink Plenty of Water

When you increase your fiber intake, you'll need to increase your water intake as well. This helps to prevent bloating and gas and regulates your bowels. Fluid needs vary based on gender, age, weight, and activity level. General guidelines suggest that adults consume 9–13 cups of water daily.

Focus on Healthy Fats

Eating healthy fats has many benefits, such as increasing high-density lipoprotein (HDL) cholesterol (considered the "good" cholesterol), absorbing fat-soluble vitamins, and reducing inflammation. Aim to include healthy fats in your meals and snacks to satisfy hunger, boost flavor, and improve mood.

Healthy fats include:

- Olives
- Avocados
- Nuts (pistachios, walnuts, almonds)
- Seeds (flax, hemp, chia)
- Fatty fish (salmon, sardines, mackerel)

Consume Enough Protein

Protein is an important nutrient for building and repairing tissue, improving enzyme and hormone production, and developing muscle, bones, skin, blood, and cartilage. It also takes a while to digest, which can make you feel full longer. Some studies suggest that eating more protein can lead to weight loss by preserving muscle mass and preventing metabolic slowdown.

Choose protein sources low in saturated fat, including white-meat chicken, eggs, turkey, fish, beans, low-fat dairy, nuts, seeds, and whole grains. Be sure to include protein sources in meals and snacks.

Supplements

Discuss your supplement intake with your healthcare provider since certain supplements can affect thyroid function and may interact with thyroid medication by reducing absorption.

Managing Symptoms

In addition to helping you lose weight or maintain a healthy weight, your diet can also help reduce various symptoms of hypothyroidism, including the following.

Bloating

Bloating is a common symptom in people with an underactive thyroid. Hypothyroidism can cause as much as a 5- to 10-pound weight gain from excess water alone. Some of that water weight gain may be in the face, causing puffiness around the eyes, fluid retention, and swelling in the hands, feet, and abdomen.

Identify triggers that can cause bloating. Foods high in sodium, such as hot dogs, pizza, certain types of bread, soups, and processed foods, can worsen fluid retention.

Increasing your fiber intake too quickly or without consuming enough water can cause bloating and gas. Research suggests that following a low-FODMAP (fermentable oligosaccharides, disaccharides, monosaccharides, and polyols) diet may ease bloating. This diet is not specific to hypothyroidism but can be helpful to people who suffer from irritable bowel syndrome (IBS) or small intestinal bacterial overgrowth (SIBO).

The low-FODMAP diet, which reduces certain carbohydrates, is not meant for all. Consult with your healthcare provider or a registered dietitian for more information.

Constipation

Consuming fiber, like beans, whole grains, and apples, can relieve constipation. Drinking adequate amounts of water also helps you maintain healthy bowel function.

Talk with your healthcare provider if your dietary changes do not help your constipation.

Fatigue

Some people with thyroid disease still note fatigue despite regulating their thyroid hormone levels. In this case, your healthcare provider may want to rule out other health conditions that may cause fatigue, such as anemia (lack of healthy red blood cells) or depression. Regular exercise, a consistent bedtime routine, and reducing sugary foods from your diet can help fight fatigue.

Proper Nutrition

Since nutritional deficiencies may worsen symptoms of thyroid disease, ensuring adequate vitamin and mineral levels is important.

Iodine

Iodine deficiency is the leading cause of thyroid dysfunction worldwide. Getting iodine from small amounts of iodized salt, seawater fish, sea vegetables (seaweed), dairy, eggs, and grains may aid in thyroid health by preventing a deficiency.

It's important not to supplement with iodine unless it's recommended by your healthcare provider, as this can cause symptoms to flare.

Vitamin D

Besides sunlight exposure, you can get vitamin D from foods like oily fish, eggs, fortified milk, and cereals. Vitamin D maintains strong bones, and research suggests it plays a role in immune system health. Some studies suggest that vitamin D deficiency is linked to thyroid dysfunction.

Vitamin B12

Research suggests that up to 40% of people with the autoimmune disease Hashimoto's thyroiditis are deficient in vitamin B12, which is found in fish, meat, dairy products, fortified cereals, and nutritional yeast. Vitamin B12 is critical for producing red blood cells and neurological function.

Selenium

Selenium is a mineral found in foods like Brazil nuts, tuna, lobster, halibut, and grass-fed beef. Early research suggests that selenium supplementation can improve the mood or well-being of those with Hashimoto's thyroiditis. This effect is more pronounced in people with deficiency or low levels at the onset.

Too much selenium is associated with gastrointestinal disease, type 2 diabetes, and cancer. Therefore, have your selenium levels checked before starting supplementation.

Foods to limit and avoid

You don't have to avoid many foods if you have hypothyroidism, but there are certain foods that may cause issues in some people with hypothyroidism.

Gluten and ultra-processed foods

Gluten is a group of proteins found in wheat, barley, triticale, and rye.

Some studies suggest that people with Hashimoto's thyroiditis may benefit from following a gluten-free diet. Other studies disagree on whether a gluten-free diet is necessary for everyone with the condition.

Additionally, people with hypothyroidism may want to limit certain foods in order to promote overall health.

For example, people with Hashimoto's thyroiditisTrusted Source have been shown to have increased markers of inflammation and oxidative stress. Oxidative stress is characterized by an excess of reactive compounds called free radicals in the body, which overwhelm the body's antioxidant defenses and can lead to cellular damage.

People with hypothyroidism may want to avoid foods that contribute to oxidative stress and inflammation, such as ultra-processed foods, foods and beverages high in added sugar, and fried foods.

In addition to contributing to oxidative stress, a diet high in these foods is linked to obesity, so cutting back on these products could also help people maintain a healthy body weight.

Goitrogens

Goitrogens are substances found in cruciferous vegetables, such as cabbage and Brussels sprouts, and soy products that may interfere with thyroid hormone production.

Most people, including those with hypothyroidism, can enjoy moderate amounts of goitrogenic foods without negatively affecting their thyroid health. Cruciferous vegetables like broccoli are actually quite low in goitrogens.

Plus, cooking goitrogenic foods reduces goitrogenic activity, making them safer for people with hypothyroidism.

That being said, it's a good idea to avoid consuming large amounts of juice made with raw cruciferous vegetables.

People with hypothyroidism may want to avoid eating large amounts of:

- cabbage
- Russian kale
- bok choy
- Brussels sprouts
- Other goitrogenic foods include soy and pearl millet.

In general, people with hypothyroidism may want to avoid eating large amounts of any goitrogenic foods.

Diet and thyroid medication

Make sure you're taking your thyroid medication on an empty stomach to promote optimal absorption. This includes avoiding beverages, foods, and supplements that could interfere with medication absorption.

Experts suggest taking thyroid medications like levothyroxine at least 30–60 minutes before breakfast or at least 3–4 hours after dinner.

Even coffee can significantly affect thyroid medication absorption, so it's important to always take your medication on an empty stomach and wait at least 30 minutes before consuming foods or beverages besides water.

It's also important to avoid taking thyroid medication within 4 hours of taking iron or calcium supplements.

People with hypothyroidism don't have to avoid many foods, but they may want to avoid consuming large amounts of goitrogenic foods and limit ultra-processed foods to promote overall health. Additionally, people with Hashimoto's thyroiditis may benefit from a gluten-free diet.

Foods to eat

Following a diet rich in nutritious foods can help improve overall health and promote healthy body weight maintenance.

Plus, a nutrient-dense diet can help reduce the risk of health conditions linked with hypothyroidism, such as heart disease, obesity, and type 2 diabetes.

A diet high in fiber can also help lower the risk of constipation, which is a common symptom of hypothyroidism.

If you have hypothyroidism, try incorporating the following nutritious foods into your diet:

- Non-starchy vegetables: greens, artichokes, zucchini, asparagus, carrots, peppers, spinach, or mushrooms
- Fruits: berries, apples, peaches, pears, grapes, citrus fruits, pineapple, or bananas
- Starchy vegetables: sweet potatoes, potatoes, peas, or butternut squash
- Fish, eggs, meat, and poultry: fish and shellfish, eggs, turkey, or chicken
- Healthy fats: olive oil, avocados, avocado oil, coconut oil, unsweetened coconut, or full fat yogurt
- Gluten-free grains: brown rice, rolled oats, quinoa, or brown rice pasta

- Seeds, nuts, and nut butters: almonds, cashews, macadamia nuts, pumpkin seeds, or natural peanut butter
- Beans and lentils: chickpeas, kidney beans, or lentils
- Dairy and nondairy substitutes: coconut milk, cashew milk, coconut yogurt, almond milk, unsweetened yogurt, or cheese
- Spices, herbs, and condiments: spices like paprika, saffron, or turmeric, fresh or dried herbs like basil or rosemary, and condiments salsa or mustard.
- Beverages: water, unsweetened tea, coffee, or sparkling water

Keep in mind that some people with hypothyroidism may benefit from avoiding gluten and other ingredients like dairy. Others may not need to cut these foods from their diet and may be able to consume gluten and dairy without an issue.

This is why it's important to develop an eating plan that works for you and your specific health needs.

If you can, work with a registered dietitian who can help identify which foods you may need to eliminate. They can also help you develop a balanced eating plan that doesn't unnecessarily cut out nutrient-rich ingredients.

1 Hypothyroidism Recipes

1.1 Berry Green Smoothie

Ingredients

1 tbsp tyrosine (sunflower seeds or flax seeds)

1 cup greens (kale, watercress, or spinach)

1/2 cup antioxidants (frozen raspberries or blueberries)

1 cup water

Directions

Place preferred tyrosine base, green base, and antioxidant base into blender.

Add water and blend until desired texture is reached.

1.2 Mixed Berry Banana Smoothie

Ingredients

100ml (1/2 cup) x Almond Milk

1 x Medium Banana

80g (3 oz) x Frozen Mixed Berries

1 x cut of spinach

1 x scoop Hemp or Pea Protein

Water as needed

Directions

Place all of the ingredients in a blender and blend until smooth

If your smoothie is too thick, add water until the desired consistency is reached. Quick and easy – Enjoy

1.3 Green Monster Smoothie

Ingredients

1 cup unsweetened almond milk

1 small banana, frozen

2 cups baby spinach

1 tablespoon chia seeds

1 scoop vanilla protein powder

8-10 cup ice cubes

Directions

Blend all of the ingredients together in a blender until smooth.

1.4 Goji Grapefruit Parsley Smoothie

Ingredients

Handful of dry goji berries that have been soaked

½ grapefruit

Handful of fresh parsley

Handful of hemp seeds

1.5 tbsps. of ground flax seed (flax seed meal)

1 tbsp of milk thistle

Handful of almonds, pecans or walnut

1 cup of filtered water

Directions

Soak the goji berries for or least two hours or overnight.

Combine all ingredients in a blender.

Blend till either very smooth or somewhat smooth if you like chunks in your smoothie.

1.5 Spinach Peach Smoothie

Ingredients

1 bunch of spinach

1 bunch dandelion

1 ripe peach

½ tsp star anise, ground

½ tsp vanilla powder or essence

2 tbsp tahini paste (ground sesame seeds)

2 tbsp flax seed, ground

1 tbsp lemon juice

2 pinches of sea salt

Directions

Throw all ingredients into a blender and blend to desired consistency.

1.6 Silky Choco-Hazelnut Smoothie

Ingredients

1 cup hazelnuts

1.5 tbsp raw cacao powder

½ cup hemp seeds

1 tsp maca powder

2 pitted dates

2 tbsp coconut butter

3 cups of water

1 tsp bee pollen – optional

Directions

Blend all ingredients on high and for long enough to get a silky texture. If using bee pollen, do not blend it but sprinkle it on top of the smoothie (otherwise it will become bitter).

1.7 Cashew Butter Green Smoothie

Ingredients

Cashew layer:

1 banana

1/4 cup cashew butter

1 tbsp chia seeds

1/4 cup unsweetened almond milk

Green layer:

1/2 banana, 1/2 avocado

1/2 cup dairy-free plain yogurt

1/4 cup unsweetened almond milk

Directions

Mix the cashew ingredients together in a blender (banana, cashew butter, chia seeds, milk) and blend until smooth.

Pour into a glass.

Rinse out the blender, but don't wash it completely (you can if you want, but it's not necessary).

Place the green ingredients together into the blender (banana, avocado, yogurt, milk) and blend until smooth.

Slowly pour the green mixture overtop the cashew butter layer. Enjoy!

1.8   Super green Basil Smoothie

Ingredients

1 small zucchini

Handful of basil

Handful of parsley

Handful of sprouts

1 carrot

2 tsp lime juice

Zest from ½ lime

¼ tsp sea salt

¼ cup of olive oil

2 cloves of garlic

½ tsp ground cumin

¼ inch ginger root

½ cup of water

Directions

Just blend it all up!

1.9   Pumpkin Smoothie

Ingredients

1½ cups lukewarm water

½ cup pumpkin puree from BPA-free can or, steamed and scooped out fresh pumpkin

¼ cup pecans/walnuts

2 tablespoons flax seed

Handful of dandelion leaves

¼ inch fresh ginger root, grated

1 tablespoon tahini

1 tablespoon coconut butter

1 date, pitted

¼ teaspoon pure vanilla extract

¼ teaspoon cinnamon

¼ teaspoon camu camu

Pinch of sea salt

Directions

Put all the ingredients in the blender and puree until silky smooth.

1.10 Turmeric Chai Latte (dairy free)

Ingredients

3 cups of water

Masala chai mix

2 teaspoons rooibos or black tea

1 large Ceylon cinnamon stick, broken to pieces

2-inch fresh ginger root, sliced

8 cardamom pods, crushed

5 cloves, crushed

1 teaspoon fennel seed

½ teaspoon black pepper corns, crushed

Other ingredients

2 pitted dates

3 tablespoons ghee or coconut butter

1 teaspoon turmeric

¼ teaspoon vanilla powder (optional)

½ teaspoon nutmeg powder (optional)

Directions

Place the water and the masala chai mix in the saucepan and bring water to a boil. Reduce the heat and simmer for 10-15 minutes. Strain and transfer to the blender. Add dates and ghee and blend on high for 1 minute. Add turmeric powder and blend again for a few seconds.

Pour to serving glasses and sprinkle with vanilla powder and nutmeg powder, if using.

1.11 Overnight Chocolate Chia Seed Pudding

Ingredients

1/4 cup cacao powder or unsweetened cocoa powder

3-5 Tbsp maple syrup

1/2 tsp ground cinnamon (optional)

1 pinch sea salt

1/2 tsp vanilla extract

1 1/2 cups Almond Breeze Almondmilk Original Unsweetened (or light coconut milk for creamier texture!)

1/2 cup chia seeds

Directions

To a small mixing bowl add cacao powder (sift first to reduce clumps), maple syrup, ground cinnamon, salt, and vanilla and whisk to combine. Then add a little dairy-free milk at a time and whisk until a paste forms. Then add remaining dairy-free milk and whisk until smooth.

Add chia seeds and whisk once more to combine. Then cover and refrigerate overnight, or at least 3-5 hours (until it's achieved a pudding-like consistency).

Leftovers keep covered in the fridge for 4-5 days, though best when fresh. Serve chilled with desired toppings, such as fruit, granola, or coconut whipped cream.

1.12 Green Plantain (Grain-Free) Pancake

Ingredients

2 medium size green or yellow plantains (if using yellow, be sure they are still firm), or 1.5lb

1 tablespoon lime juice

¼ cup of coconut oil, ghee or lard, melted

Generous pinch of sea salt

2 teaspoons ghee or coconut oil, divided

Filling - sweet option (for 2)

1 cup mixed berries

2 tablespoons coconut butter

1 teaspoon lime juice

1 teaspoon vanilla essence

Pinch of sea salt

Filling - savory option (for 2)

1 avocado

2 strips of bacon, cooked

Handful of arugula leaves

Handful of sprouts

Whipped Coconut Cream (optional)

Coconut milk can, 13.66 oz

½ teaspoon vanilla essence

3 drops of liquid stevia

Directions

Peel and slice up the plantain.

Combine the plantain, lime juice, coconut oil and salt in a blender and blend until smooth. Add water if you need to help the blender blades work the batter.

Melt 1 teaspoon of ghee in a ceramic non-stick skillet. If you use a cast iron skillet, the pancake might stick.

Spread half the mixture in the skillet. Make the second pancake in the second skillet or after this one is done.

Cover and leave an opening for the water to evaporate.

Cook on low medium heat for 10 minutes or until the top is dry, then flip it.

Cook for another 2 to 3 minutes or until browned.

Serve with either sweet or savory filling.

1.13 Fruit & Coconut Yogurt Parfait

Ingredients

1 cup unsweetened coconut milk yogurt (or Greek yogurt)

2 tablespoons sunflower seeds

2 tablespoons shredded coconut (optional)

Dash cinnamon

¼ cup berries of choice

1 teaspoon stevia to sweeten (optional)

Directions

In a bowl or glass add ½ cup coconut milk yogurt.

Top with 1 tablespoon sunflower seeds, coconut, cinnamon and 1/8 cup berries.

Top with ½ cup coconut milk yogurt, 1 tablespoon sunflower seeds, coconut, cinnamon and 1/8 cup berries.

Top with optional stevia and serve.

Tip: If you're strapped for time, blend it all up in smoothie form, adding a little coconut or almond milk to thin if needed.

1.14 Coconut Flour Porridge

Ingredients

2 tablespoons coconut flour

2 tablespoons golden flax meal

3/4 cup water

Pinch of salt

1 large egg, beaten

2 teaspoons butter or ghee

1 tablespoon heavy cream or coconut milk

1 tablespoon Sukrin Gold or your favorite sweetener

Directions

Measure the first four ingredients into a small pot over medium heat and stir. When it begins to simmer, turn it down to medium-low and whisk until it begins to thicken.

Remove the coconut flour porridge from heat and add the beaten egg, a half at a time, while whisking continuously. Place back on the heat and continue to whisk until the porridge thickens.

Remove from the heat and continue to whisk for about 30 seconds before adding the butter, cream and sweetener.

Garnish with your favorite toppings.

1.15 Banana Pancakes

Ingredients

One banana

One egg*

Extra virgin coconut oil

Strawberries for garnishing

Directions

Blend banana and egg in mixer until batter consistency achieved (30 sec – 1 minute). Melt coconut oil in pan. Pour batter into pan.

Cook for 2-3 minutes and then flip cooking for additional 1-2 minutes

Cut strawberries in half to garnish

TIP: putting a cover over the pan will even out the cooking process and help prevent destruction of pancake upon flipping

1.16 Coconut Flour Pancakes With Blueberry Maple Syrup

Ingredients

1/4 cup coconut flour

1/4 teaspoon baking soda

2 tablespoons your favorite natural nut butter of choice

2 eggs, slightly beaten

½ tablespoon honey or maple syrup

1/2 medium banana, mashed

¼ cup unsweetened vanilla almond milk

For the syrup:

2/3 cup wild organic blueberries

2 tablespoons pure maple syrup

Directions

In large bowl whisk together coconut flour and baking soda; set aside.

In a separate medium bowl, mix together the nut butter, eggs, honey, banana and almond milk together until smooth and well combined. Add wet ingredients to flour mixture and mix together.

1.17 Banana Breakfast Pancakes

Ingredients

1 medium-sized banana, peeled

2 x 15ml tbsp finely shredded dried coconut

1 x 15ml tbsp coconut flour

1 tsp coconut oil

Blueberries and maple syrup, to serve

Directions

Heat the coconut oil in a non-stick frying pan.

Mash the banana in a bowl, until it's soft and runny. Stir in the dried coconut and the coconut flour to form a thick dough, a bit like a soft biscuit dough. Bananas can vary, so add a little more coconut flour if you need it.

Take a heaped tablespoonful of the dough and drop into the coconut oil. Spread the pancake out with the back of the spoon, dipping it in the oil in the pan, if it sticks. Cook for 1-2 minutes on the first side and then flip - it should be slightly golden - and continue to cook for about 2 minutes on the other side.

When cooked through, serve the pancakes while they're still hot, with a small drizzle of maple syrup and a handful of blueberries on the side.

1.18 Banana Muffins

Ingredients

1 & 1/4 cup almond flour

1/4 cup flax seed flour (optional)

2 teaspoons baking powder

1/4 teaspoon baking soda

1 teaspoon cinnamon

1/2 cup unsweetened apple sauce

2 eggs*

3 ripe mashed bananas

Optional-may choose to add one or more of the following

1/2 cup shaved coconut

1/2 cup blueberries

1/2 cup walnuts

1/4 cup poppy seeds

1 tablespoon unsweetened cocoa powder + 1/4 cup honey

Directions

Mix all ingredients

Bake for 45 minutes to 1 hour at 350 degrees Fahrenheit or until tops of muffins are lightly browned, one hour if baking banana bread.

1.19 Carrot Orange Muffins

Ingredients

Wet ingredients

3 tablespoons ground flaxseed

⅓ Cup hot water

2 cups grated carrots, lightly packed

1 cup unsweetened apple sauce

½ cup coconut oil, melted

1 orange, peeled and cut to chunks

¼ cup coconut nectar (where to buy)

1 tablespoon vanilla extract

10 drops stevia (optional)

Dry ingredients

1.5 cups brown rice flour

1 cup teff flour

2 tablespoons ground cinnamon

2 teaspoons baking powder

1 teaspoon baking soda

½ teaspoons sea salt

Directions

Preheat the oven to 375F.

Combine the flax seed and water and set aside for about 10 minutes.

Mix all the dry ingredients in one bowl.

Mix all the wet ingredients in another, larger bowl, including the flax seed slurry.

Add the dry ingredients to the larger bowl with the wet ingredients and mix gently to combine them. Do not over mix.

Line the muffin form with muffin cups and dish out the batter to each cup.

Bake for 25 minutes or until the tops are firm to touch.

1.20 Savory Oatmeal Sweet Potatoes

Ingredients

½ cup red peppers, diced

¼ cup rolled oats

¾ cups water

½ small sweet potato, diced

1 scallion, chopped

1 tsp coconut oil

1 tbsp maple syrup

2 slices of bacon

Optional ingredients for garnish:

¼ cup walnuts, chopped

¼ cup cranberries

1 tbsp coconut flakes

Directions

In a large skillet, heat 1 tbsp coconut oil over medium heat.

Add the red peppers, sweet potatoes, and sauté for 10 mins until the sweet potatoes begin to soften.

Add half of the scallion and cook for another 5 mins.

Next cook the bacon according to desired crispiness.

Next bring ¾ cups of water to a boil and stir in ¼ cups of rolled oats. Reduce the heat to a simmer, continue to stir frequently for 5-10 mins or until the oats are tender and the water has evaporated.

For extra sweetness, stir in 1 tbsp of maple syrup

Add the red pepper & sweet potato mixture, bacon, and the rest of the chopped scallion.

Garnish with walnuts, cranberries, and coconut flakes and enjoy!

1.21 Quinoa Stir Fry

Ingredients

1 onion, chopped

2 tbsps. coconut oil

1 cup of quinoa (white or red)

2 cups of water

2 roasted peppers (red or yellow)

2 cups of mushrooms, chopped

4 carrots, chopped

1 bunch of kale, chard or bok choy

1 yellow squash

1 tsp cumin seeds

Directions

Soak the quinoa grains for 5-10 minutes.

Change the water and cook it till soft and fluffy, about 15 minutes.

In a large pan or wok, fry the onion in coconut oil till translucent.

Add chopped mushrooms and cook till onions and mushrooms turn brown.

Add carrots and cook for 5-7 minutes.

Add yellow squash and roasted peppers (for quick roasting, hold the pepper in kitchen tongs over a stove fire and keep turning the pepper till all sides are soft and the skin is blackened) and cook for another few minutes.

In a separate small pan, roast cumin seeds in a dry pan over low to medium heat, shaking the pan frequently to roll the seeds around until they are aromatic and a darker shade.

Once quinoa is cooked, combine it with the vegetables and cumin and cook through another minute.

Serve warm.

Note: You can make it for a few morning servings ahead and just warm it up gently each time. One trick not to overcook food is to cook the food you want for later to no more than 80%. This way when you are reheating it, you are not overcooking it.

1.22 Almond Flour Zucchini Apple Pancakes

Ingredients

1 small zucchini, grated

1 small apple, grated

1 cup almond flour

½ teaspoon baking powder (skip if you are doing GAPS)

½ teaspoon sea salt

2-3 tablespoons almond butter (you can use any nut butter, really)

3 sprigs of fresh thyme, chopped

3 eggs

1 tablespoon honey (raw, unheated) or maple syrup (use honey if you are doing GAPS)

2 tablespoons of coconut oil

Directions

Combine apples, zucchini, thyme, honey and almond butter in one bowl

Combine flour, salt and baking powder in another bowl

Beat the eggs, just slightly

Combine all ingredients

Heat up the coconut oil and fry pancakes, about 5 minutes per side, without burning.

Serve them with yoghurt and fresh fruit or your favorite jam.

1.23 Sweet Potato Fritters

Ingredients

3 cups grated sweet potato (about 1 large sweet potato)

4 eggs whisked

2 tsp. paprika

Salt and pepper

Butter/ghee for the pan

Directions

Squeeze out any excess juice from the grated sweet potato and place in to a bowl. Add the eggs, paprika, salt and pepper and mix well.

In a fry pan on medium heat melt some butter.

Use a 1/4 cup to scoop out fritter batter, carefully form in to a fritter with your hands and place in to the fry pan.

Cook for 5 minutes, flip, press down with a spatula, then cook for a further 5 minutes. Continue to do this with all the fritter batter, it will make about 10-12 fritters.

Serve with mashed avocado, lemon and a drizzle of olive oil! Yum!

1.24 Sweet potato Hash {Greek Style} With Feta Cheese & Eggs

Ingredients

2 medium California sweet potatoes {~ 4 cups shredded}

2 tablespoons extra virgin olive oil

1 medium onion finely chopped

4 cups chopped baby spinach

1 tablespoon dried Greek seasoning*

1/4 teaspoon sea salt or to taste

Fresh ground black pepper to taste

4 eggs**

4 ounces feta cheese

Fresh oregano for garnish optional

Directions

Prepare the veggies: Peel the sweet potatoes, then shred them with a food processor, and set aside, then chop the onions by hand or in a food processor, and set aside. Chop the baby spinach, and set aside.

Heat the olive oil over medium in a 12-inch cast iron, or other, skillet. Add the shredded sweet potatoes and toss to coat in the oil. Cook the sweet potatoes over medium for about 5 minutes, tossing regularly so they don't burn. Add the chopped onion and cook for an additional 4 minutes, then add the chopped spinach and cook for 1-2 minutes, or until wilted.

Stir in the Greek seasoning, sea salt and ground black pepper to taste.

Spread the veggie mixture evenly across the pan, and make 4 holes in the veggies. Next, crack one egg in each hole, and cook for ~ 2 minutes, then place a lid over the pan and cook for an additional 3 minutes, or until eggs are cooked to your liking.

Remove skillet from heat, and top with crumbled feta cheese and fresh oregano for garnish before dividing in to 4 servings.

1.25 Coconut Macadamia Granola

Ingredients

4 c rolled oats, preferably gluten-free

2 c unsweetened shredded coconut

1 c sliced almonds

1 c chopped macadamia nuts, roasted, unsalted (or salted and adjust salt)

1 c pumpkin seeds, unsalted

1/2 c sesame seeds, preferably raw, unhulled *

1/2 c chia seeds

1/2 c unrefined coconut oil (105 g)

1 c honey (340 g)

1/2 c maple syrup (170 g)

1/2 tsp. cardamom

1/4 tsp. cinnamon

1/4 tsp. ginger

1/2 tsp. vanilla extract

1 tsp. fine sea salt (or to taste)

Directions

Arrange two oven racks in upper and lower third of oven and preheat to 275 F. Line 2 large rimmed baking sheets with parchment, or grease with coconut oil.

In a large mixing bowl combine first 8 (dry) ingredients and set aside.

In a medium saucepan combine coconut oil, honey, syrup, and spices. Place over medium flame and heat, stirring, just until coconut oil is melted and mixture is runny.

Remove from heat and stir in vanilla extract.

Pour wet mixture over dry mixture and toss to coat. Sprinkle in sea salt and toss again.

Spread granola evenly on baking sheets and place in oven. Bake 1 hour, stirring granola and alternating sheet pans every 15 minutes for even baking. Do not over bake.

If necessary, break up any large clumps while still warm, and set aside to cool. Granola will lose its stickiness as it cools. Store in an airtight container or plastic bag. Granola will keep for several weeks.

1.26 Chocolate Cherry Almond Granola

Ingredients

1/4 c cacao powder (or sub. cocoa powder)

3 c rolled oats, preferably gluten-free

1 c sliced almonds

1/2 c hulled hemp seeds (or sub. sesame seeds)

1/2 tsp. fine sea salt

1/2 tsp. cinnamon

1/3 c unrefined coconut oil

1/3 c maple syrup

1/4 tsp. vanilla extract

1/4 tsp. almond extract

3 tbsp. raw turbinado sugar

1 tsp. flake sea salt, like Maldon (or less to taste)

1 c sweetened dried cherries

2 oz chopped semi-sweet chocolate

Directions

Preheat oven to 275.

In a large mixing bowl, combine cacao, oats, almonds, hemp (or sesame seeds), fine sea salt, and cinnamon. Stir to combine.

In a small pan over low heat, combine coconut oil, maple syrup, vanilla extract, and almond extract. Heat, stirring, just until fat is melted. Pour mixture over dry ingredients and stir to combine. Spread mixture on a rimmed, parchment-lined baking sheet and place in center of oven. Bake 30 minutes. Remove from oven and sprinkle with turbinado sugar and flake sea salt, stir gently and return to oven. Bake 20 minutes more. Remove granola from oven, and stir in dried cherries-- this will help the cherries adhere a bit before the granola fully dries as it cools. Finally, sprinkle with chopped chocolate but do not stir-- this will also help the chocolate adhere. Set aside to cool, 2 hours. Store in an airtight container for up to 1 month.

1.27 Cranberry Zinger

Ingredients

1 1/4 c fresh or frozen cranberries

2 medium oranges, peeled and thickly sliced, seeds removed

1 ripe pear, peeled, cored, and cut into chunks

1 c crushed ice

1 tbsp. maple syrup

1 1/2 inch piece ginger, peeled and sliced

Directions

Combine all ingredients in a blender, and blend at high speed until smooth.

1.28 Basted Eggs Over Sausage & Pepper Hash

Ingredients

2 tsp. ghee

1 small yellow onion, diced

2 cloves garlic, minced

3/4 c sliced button mushrooms

2 large links chicken-apple sausage, diced

1 medium red bell pepper, diced

1/2 c grated cheddar cheese

4 eggs

1 tbsp. chopped chives or green onion, for garnish

1/3 c fresh diced tomato, for garnish

salt, pepper, and cayenne to taste

Directions

First make sure you have a medium-large skillet with a tight fitting lid. Place over medium-high heat and add ghee.

Once ghee has melted and pan is hot, add the onion, garlic, mushrooms, and sausage. Cook, stirring, until the onions have begun to soften and the mix is really talking to you (sizzle sizzle sizzle!).

Add the peppers and continue to cook until the mixture is beginning to brown in spots.

Taste and season the mixture with salt, pepper, and cayenne if desired.

Reduce heat to medium-low. Use the back of a spoon to make 4 shallow, egg-sized divots in the hash. Sprinkle on the cheese and then crack the eggs into the divots. Cover with tight fitting lid.

All that steam is what's going to cook your eggs. At this point the pan should still be talking to you, but more quietly (sizzle...sizzle...sizzle...). If it's too loud, reduce your heat. Be patient with this part, so you don't burn the bottom. The eggs can take a while to reach the desired degree of doneness. Take a quick peek, but put the lid right back on to keep all that hot steam in. Test the eggs by touching the yolk for firmness. Don't be shy. The sunny-looking eggs might appear 'easy', even when they're hard.

Once the eggs have reached your preferred degree of doneness, remove from heat, and sprinkle with chives and diced tomato. Use a spatula to scoop portions from pan to plate. Enjoy!

1.29 Mini Mushroom and Sausage Quiches

Ingredients

8 ounces sausage, turkey, breakfast, removed from casing and crumbled into small pieces

1 teaspoon oil, olive, extra-virgin

8 ounces mushrooms, sliced

1/4 cup scallions (green onions), sliced

1/4 cup cheese, Swiss, shredded

1 teaspoon pepper, black ground, freshly ground

5 large eggs

3 large egg whites

1 cup milk, low-fat (1%)

Directions

Position rack in center of oven; preheat to 325°F. Coat a non-stick muffin tin generously with cooking spray.

Heat a large non-stick skillet over medium-high heat. Add sausage and cook until golden brown, 6 to 8 minutes. Transfer to a bowl to cool. Add oil to the pan. Add mushrooms and cook, stirring often, until golden brown, 5 to 7 minutes. Transfer mushrooms to the bowl with the sausage. Let cool for 5 minutes. Stir in scallions, cheese, and pepper.

Whisk eggs, egg whites, and milk in a medium bowl. Divide the egg mixture evenly among the prepared muffin cups. Sprinkle a heaping tablespoon of the sausage mixture into each cup.

Bake until the tops are just beginning to brown, 25 minutes. Let cool on a wire rack for 5 minutes. Place a rack on top of the pan, flip it over and turn the quiches out onto the rack. Turn upright and let cool completely.

1.30 Lamb Hash with Carrot & Celery Root

Ingredients

1 lb ground AIP lamb sausage, recipe below

1 medium celery root, peeled and diced (1/3-inch cubes)

1 lb carrots, peeled and diced (1/3-inch cubes)

1/2 tsp. sea salt, or more to taste

1/8 tsp. ground cinnamon

1/4 tsp. turmeric

1 tbsp. maple syrup

Freshly ground black pepper, optional (see note 2)

Directions

In a large skillet over medium-high heat, brown the lamb sausage until crisp in spots, 7 - 10 minutes. Remove sausage with a slotted spoon and set aside, leaving about 2 tablespoons of rendered lamb fat in the pan. Discard remaining fat or save for other uses.

Add diced celery root, carrots, and sea salt to skillet, and cook 5 minutes over medium-high heat, stirring occasionally. Add cinnamon, turmeric, and maple syrup, and cook, stirring, 5 minutes more or until well-browned.

Return lamb to skillet, cook 1 more minute. Taste and adjust seasoning if necessary.

1.31 Herbed Lamb Sausage

Ingredients

3 lb ground lamb, preferably grass fed and pasture raised

2 tsp. sea salt

4 large cloves garlic, minced

1/2 c chopped parsley (fresh)

1 tbsp. chopped rosemary (fresh)

1 tbsp. chopped thyme (fresh)

1 tbsp. chopped mint (fresh)

Directions

In a large mixing bowl, combine all ingredients, and mix together with clean hands until all herbs and seasonings are dispersed.

At this point, you may wish to set a portion of the sausage aside for additional meals like Lamb Hash, or Lamb Meatballs en Brodo.

For breakfast patties, roll into golf-ball sized rounds, and flatten to 1/2 - 2/3 inch thick patties. Heat a large skillet over medium-high heat, and add patties to pan, working in batches to avoid over-crowding and ensure a nice brown crust. Cook 4 - 5 minutes per side or until browned and slightly-pink in the center. Remove from pan, let cool, and store as desired in fridge and/or freezer.

A few tips

Keeping your hands wet while forming patties, burgers, or meatballs will keep the meat from sticking to them. Keep a bowl of cool water nearby to dip your hands in.

To ensure a moist and juicy sausage patty, avoid overcooking, especially if you plan to freeze and reheat them later. Make it 5 minutes per side, maintaining a slightly-pink center.

Lamb renders the most delicious fat as it sizzles and browns. No additional oil is needed, but a splatter guard may come in handy.

1.32 Eggnog – Dairy & Egg free

Ingredients

1 ½ cups filtered water

⅓ heaping cup pecans

1 tablespoon maple syrup or raw honey

1 teaspoon vanilla extract

½ teaspoon freshly ground nutmeg

¼ teaspoon ground Ceylon cinnamon

⅛ teaspoon ground cloves

Pinch of sea salt

½ ounce rum, optional

Directions

Place all the ingredients in the blender and whizz until smooth.

Serve warm or cold.

1.33 Simple Bone Broth

Ingredients

1 medium, white onion

2 medium carrots, chopped

3-4 stalks celery

1 leek, halved

7 garlic cloves, smashed

5 lb. bones (from pastured, grass-fed meat – see "A note on bones")

2 tbsp. apple cider vinegar

Herbs/spices:

1 tsp. cracked whole black peppercorns

6 sprigs parsley

6 sprigs thyme

2 bay leaves

Salt to taste

1 tsp. turmeric powder

Directions

Cut onion, carrots, celery and leek into chunks and add to a crockpot with the bones. Add smashed garlic and apple cider vinegar.

Fill the crockpot to the brim with filtered water.

Cook broth anywhere from 24-48 hours on "low" in the crockpot (If working on a stovetop, you'll want to keep it on a very low simmer, covered, for the same amount of time. If you don't feel comfortable leaving the stove on at night, turn it to the very lowest setting, then turn it back up in the morning.)

When you have about 2 hours left, add herbs/spices and make sure they're covered with liquid.

After the allotted time, turn the heat off and let the broth cool down until it's safe to handle.

Strain the liquid into a large bowl and discard all solids. From here, you can transfer your broth into smaller containers and fridge or freeze. Keep bone broth for up to one week in the fridge or freeze for up to six months.

1.34 Ginger-Chicken Noodle Soup

Ingredients

1 pound chicken, thighs skinless, boneless, cut into 1-inch pieces

1 tablespoon oil, cooking

2 medium carrots cut into thin bite-size sticks

3 cans broth, chicken, less sodium 14 ounces each

1 cup water

2 tablespoons vinegar, rice

1 tablespoon soy sauce, less sodium

2 1/2 teaspoons ginger, fresh

1/4 teaspoon pepper, black, ground

2 ounces rice noodles, dried

6 ounces pea pods, frozen, thawed, and halved diagonally

Directions

In a Dutch oven, cook chicken, half at a time, in hot oil just until browned. Drain fat. Return all chicken to Dutch oven. Add carrots, broth, water, vinegar, soy sauce, ginger, and pepper. Bring to boiling; reduce heat and simmer, covered, 20 minutes.

Return to boil. Add noodles. Simmer, uncovered, 8 to 10 minutes or until noodles are tender, adding pea pods the last 1 to 2 minutes. If desired serve with additional soy sauce.

1.35 Split Pea Soup with Smoked Ham

Ingredients

1 tbsp. avocado oil, or heat-stable cooking fat of choice

1 small yellow onion, finely diced

3 cloves garlic, minced

1 medium shallot, minced

1 medium leek, white part only, finely diced

3 to 4 medium carrots, peeled, medium dice

3 celery ribs, medium dice

4 c chicken stock, preferably homemade

2 c water

2 c dried split peas (green or yellow, but not both—they cook at different rates)

2 c diced smoked ham (NOT honeyed), preferably nitrate-free

2 bay leaves

1 tsp. dried thyme

1 tsp. dried marjoram

Freshly ground black pepper and salt, to taste

Directions

Cover the split peas with plenty of fresh, filtered water and soak 7 hours or overnight. Drain and rinse.

Place a large soup pot over medium heat. Add the oil, onion, garlic, shallot, leek, carrots, celery, and a splash of chicken stock. Saute the vegetables, stirring occasionally, 5 – 10 minutes or until slightly softened.

Add chicken stock, water, soaked split peas, smoked ham, bay leaves, thyme and marjoram. Stir to combine. Bring to a boil, reduce heat, and simmer approx. 1 1/2 hours, stirring occasionally. The soup is done when the peas are tender and beginning to disintegrate and thicken the soup.

Taste the soup before seasoning with additional salt and pepper, as some chicken broths, and some ham add sufficient salt on their own.

1.36 Tomato, Sausage & Fennel Soup

Ingredients

1 lb sweet Italian sausage

2 tbsp. extra virgin olive oil

1 small onion (or large shallot), diced small

1 medium fennel bulb, diced small

4 cloves garlic, minced

1 large or 2 medium carrots, peeled and diced small

3 -4 stalks celery, diced small

1 1/4 tsp. ground fennel seed

2 tsp. chopped fresh thyme

4 c chicken stock, preferably homemade

One 28-oz. can whole peeled tomatoes, preferably San Marzano

Sea salt and freshly ground pepper, to taste

Directions

Place Italian sausage in a large (5-quart) soup pot over medium-high heat. Cook until browned and most liquid has evaporated. Remove from pot, drain and discard drippings, and set aside.

Add olive oil to pot over medium heat. Add fennel, garlic, onion, carrots, and celery, and cook 10 - 15 minutes or until carrots are tender. Feel free to add a splash of chicken stock to speed the process along with steam and/or prevent browning.

Add ground fennel and fresh thyme and stir to combine. Pour in chicken stock and bring to a simmer.

Meanwhile, place tomatoes in a blender and process to your desired consistency. Add to soup pot along with cooked sausage. Season with salt and pepper and simmer, covered, for 30 minutes or until flavors have melded. Taste and adjust seasoning as desired.

1.37 Orange Velvet Soup

Ingredients

2 medium onions, roughly chopped

1/4 c organic unrefined coconut oil

1/2 c cream sherry (optional)

1 1/2 lb carrots, peeled and roughly chopped

4 c chicken stock, preferably homemade

Pinch freshly grated nutmeg

14 fl oz can coconut milk

2 medium oranges, juice only

1/2 medium lime, juice only

2 inch piece fresh ginger root, peeled and minced

1 tsp. fine sea salt, or to taste

Dash white pepper, or to taste

Garnish: sliced green onion and/or toasted coconut chips

Directions

In a large soup pot over medium heat, saute onions in coconut oil until soft, about 10 minutes. Add sherry (optional), and simmer 5 minutes more or until it doesn't smell so boozy.

Add carrots, chicken stock, and nutmeg, and bring to a boil. Reduce heat to a simmer, cover and cook until carrots are tender, 20 to 30 minutes.

Add coconut milk and return to a simmer. Remove from heat and add orange juice, lime juice, and ginger.

Working in batches, carefully blend hot soup with regular* (see note) or immersion blender until smooth and velvety. Season to taste with salt and white pepper. Garnish with green onion and/or toasted coconut chips and serve.

1.38 Thai Chicken Soup with Coconut Milk

Ingredients

2 stalks lemongrass, or 1/4 cup prepared lemongrass paste (sometimes available in the produce section, refrigerated), or zest of 1 lemon

4 c chicken broth, preferably homemade

1 lb boneless, skinless chicken breasts, thinly sliced

1/2 yellow onion, thinly sliced into 1-inch-long pieces

2 c thinly sliced crimini mushrooms

5 lime leaves, or zest of 1 lime

1 [3-inch] piece galangal or fresh ginger root, cut into coins

2 large roma tomatoes

1 can coconut milk

2 to 4 tbsp. fresh squeezed lime juice (from 1 to 2 limes), or to taste

2 to 3 tbsp. fish sauce** (see note), or to taste

Sambal oelek, sriracha, or hot sauce, to taste

1 tsp. brown sugar, packed

2/3 c chopped fresh cilantro

1/4 c thinly sliced green onion

Directions

If using fresh lemon grass, cut lower half of stalk into 1-inch pieces, and discard tops.

In a large (5 quart) pot bring chicken broth to a boil. Add lemongrass, chicken breast, onion, mushrooms, and lime leaves and galangal or ginger coins. If substituting lemon and/or lime zest, do not add yet. Reduce heat and let simmer 5 – 7 minutes or until chicken is cooked through.

To peel and seed the tomatoes: use a small paring knife to remove the stem from the tomatoes, and then cut an X in the skin on the opposite end of the tomatoes. Add to broth and let simmer 1 minute, or until skins have begun to split and peel away. Remove from broth and let rest until cool enough to handle. Remove skin– it should pull away easily. Cut in half and with your fingertips, remove and discard seeds. Dice the tomato flesh into 1/4 inch cubes, and add to soup.

Reduce heat to medium. Add coconut milk, lime juice, fish sauce, chili paste or hot sauce, and brown sugar to soup. If substituting lemon and/or lime zest, add now. Stir to combine until soup is heated through* (see note).

Taste and adjust seasonings, adding more fish sauce, lime juice, brown sugar, or chilies as needed to reach the perfect salty/sour/sweet/spicy balance. Ladle into bowls. Garnish with fresh cilantro and green onion, and serve.

1.39 Pumpkin Soup

Ingredients

500grams pumpkin

2 whole onions (skin on)

1 whole knob of garlic (skin on)

Sprinkle with salt and pepper

Directions

Cut the pumpkin into wedges and chop the skin off

Cut into rough pieces. The larger the size, the longer they will take to cook.

Bake on a tray lined with non-stick baking paper at 180 degree Celsius oven for approximately 30-40 mins, until the pumpkin is nice and soft.

Remove from the oven.

Get a large saucepan ready on the stove to prepare the soup.

Squeeze out the onion from their skins into the saucepan. Do the same with the knob of garlic and discard the skins. Place pumpkin into the saucepan.

Add 1.5 Litres of chicken or vegetable stock and bring to boil.

Let boil for 5 mins. Remove from the heat and blend with a stick blender until smooth. Serve and enjoy!

1.40 Yummy Kale Salad

Ingredients

1 cup of chopped kale

6 diced heart of palm

6 chopped radishes

1/4 cup of coconut flakes

Juice of one lemon

1/4 cup of coconut milk

Directions

Toss together and serve cold.

1.41 Roasted Beet & Carrot Salad with Herbs

Salad Ingredients:

1 bunch small beets with greens attached

1 tablespoon olive oil, divided

2 medium carrots, cut into 1-inch pieces

2 cups salad greens

1 cooked chicken breast, shredded or cubed

2 teaspoons golden flax seed

2 teaspoons sesame seeds

2 tablespoons fresh parsley, roughly chopped

2 teaspoons fresh thyme

Herb Vinaigrette Ingredients:

3 tablespoons olive oil

1 ½ tablespoons lemon juice

1 tablespoon fresh parsley, roughly chopped

1 teaspoon fresh thyme, roughly chopped

1 teaspoon fresh rosemary, roughly chopped

½ teaspoon ground sea salt

Directions

Preheat oven to 375 degrees.

Chop the greens off the beets, and wash them well.

Wash the baby beets. Place the beets on parchment paper, and drizzle with 2 teaspoons of olive oil.

Seal the parchment up, place in a shallow roasting pan and bake for 30-40 minutes, or until fork tender.

Toss the carrots with remaining olive oil, and place in a shallow roasting pan. Bake for 25-30 minutes, or until fork tender.

While the vegetables are baking, bring a medium saucepan of salted water to a boil.

Blanch the beet greens for 1 minute, or until bright green. Shock them in a bowl of cold water with lots of ice cubes.

Dry the beet greens with paper towels, or in a salad spinner. Roughly chop the greens.

When the beets are cool enough to handle, gently remove their skins with paper towels. Cut off the root end of the beets.

Vinaigrette Instructions:

Whisk all of the ingredients together in a small bowl.

To Assemble:

Place the salad greens on a platter, and top with beet greens, shredded chicken, beets, roasted carrots, flax seeds, sesame seeds, parsley and thyme.

Drizzle the salad with the herb vinaigrette. Serve immediately and enjoy!

1.42 Roasted Radish & Seaweed Salad

Ingredients

2 bunches radishes (about 12-15 radishes total)

¼ cup dried arame

2 scallions, chopped

2 ½ teaspoons olive oil

1 teaspoon rice wine vinegar

1 teaspoon fish sauce

Directions

Slice the roots and green tops off the radishes. The greens can be saved for another use. Slice larger radishes in quarters, medium ones in half, and leave smaller ones whole.

Heat the oven to 375°. Toss the radishes with 1 ½ teaspoons of the olive oil and bake for 30 minutes on parchment paper, stirring halfway through.

Meanwhile, boil the kettle. Place the arame in a heat proof glass or ceramic bowl and cover with hot water. Let it sit for at least 15 minutes before draining.

After the radishes are cooked, toss them with the drained arame, the remaining 1 teaspoon olive oil, rice wine vinegar, and fish sauce. Top with the sliced scallions.

This salad can last in the fridge for up to four days, but is best enjoyed warm.

1.43 Quick Sauerkraut Salad

Ingredients

1 cup lacto-fermented sauerkraut

1 teaspoon cumin seeds, roasted

½ cup broccoli sprouts

½ avocado, sliced

1 medium carrot, grated

1 teaspoon black sesame seeds (optional)

Directions

Combine sauerkraut and cumin seeds.

Add all other ingredients into a serving bowl. Sprinkle sesame seeds if using.

1.44 Greek Yogurt Tuna Salad

Ingredients

1/4 cup plain Greek yogurt

1 tbsp mayo (spicy mustard would work fabulous!)

1 5 oz can of tuna

1 small apple, diced

2 stalks celery, diced

1 tsp chopped onion

1/4 tsp garlic salt

Salt & pepper

Lemon juice

Directions

Chop the apple and celery. Add to a bowl

Drain tuna and add it to the bowl.

Add 1/4 cup of Greek yogurt and 1 tbsp of mayo to the bowl.

Add spices, salt & pepper, and lemon juice.

Mix thoroughly and serve in pitas!

This tuna salad is sensational microwaved too, if you want something warm.

1.45 Zucchini and Anchovy Quick Salad

Ingredients

1 large zucchini, grated to slices

1 can anchovies or sardines, mashed with a fork

⅓ Bunch of dill, chopped

2 tablespoons of olive oil

Juice of 1 lemon

Sea salt

Directions

Beat together olive oil, lemon juice and sea salt into a nice vinaigrette.

Combine zucchini, anchovies (or sardines) and dill.

Pour the vinaigrette over the zucchini slides.

Mix it all together and voila!

1.46 Brown Rice Salad with Shrimp & Avocado

Ingredients

5 c cooked brown rice

1 lb raw medium shrimp, peeled and deveined

1 tbsp. minced fresh ginger

2 tbsp. rice wine (Mirin) or sake

2 small ripe avocados

Juice of 1/2 lemon

1 c quartered and sliced English cucumber

1/4 c sliced green onion

1 lemon, quartered for garnish

For The Dressing:

2 tbsp. Tamari or soy sauce

2 tbsp. seasoned rice vinegar

1 tbsp. sugar

1 tbsp. lemon juice (approx. 1/2 lemon)

1 1/2 tbsp. rice wine (Mirin) or sake

1 1/2 tbsp. toasted sesame oil

1/4 tsp. fine sea salt

Directions

If you haven't already, cook the brown rice according to package instructions. Spread the rice on a sheet pan to cool. This dish tastes best if the rice is room temp when mixed, rather than warm.

In a small bowl combine the shrimp, minced ginger, and 2 tablespoons Mirin. Toss to coat and set aside.

In another small bowl combine dressing ingredients. Whisk until salt and sugar are completely dissolved and set aside.

In a large pot bring 2 quarts water to a rolling boil. Add shrimp and marinade and boil until shrimp are cooked through and opaque, about 2 to 3 minutes. Drain in a colander and set aside to cool.

Slice avocado and squeeze with the juice of 1/2 lemon. Set aside.

In a large mixing bowl combine rice, shrimp, and cucumber, dressing and green onion. Toss lightly to combine. Taste and adjust seasonings.

Divide the salad among plates, top with avocado slices, garnish with lemon wedges, and serve.

Optional Add-Ins:

Fresh parsley, fresh cilantro, chopped pickled ginger.

1.47 Lentil and Green Pea Salad

Ingredients

1 cup frozen peas

7 oz. fresh mushrooms, sliced

½ c onion, diced

3 cups cooked lentils (no/low sodium)

½ red bell pepper, diced

3 tbsp dry parsley flakes

2 tsp ground cumin

2 tbsp white wine vinegar

2 tbsp lemon juice

Black pepper (to taste)

4 cups spinach

2 tbsp flaxseeds, ground

Directions

Begin by adding the frozen peas to a medium stovetop pan and turn to medium-high heat. Stir frequently to prevent sticking and burning. When the green peas are warm, add the fresh mushrooms and onions.

Continue to cook the peas, onion and mushrooms on medium heat until the mushrooms start to release their juice. Then add the rest of the ingredients except the spinach and flax. Heat the mixture until it's thoroughly warmed.

One serving of this recipe is 2 cups of spinach topped with half of the lentil mixture and half the flax. Enjoy warm or cold.

1.48 Chickpea & Bulgur Salad

Ingredients

2/3 cup dry bulgur

1 can chickpeas, drained (no/low sodium)

2 cups water

1 cucumber

1 red bell pepper

1 tomato

1 cup fresh parsley

2 spring onions

1 tsp garlic

Black pepper, to taste

2 tbsp white wine vinegar

1 tsp prepared mustard

1 tbsp soy sauce

2 tbsp lemon juice

1 tbsp ground flaxseeds

Extra greens, to serve

Directions

In a medium bowl, soak the bulgur in the water until hydrated. Soak it for at least an hour and up to 24 hours. When the bulgur is fully hydrated, drain the bulgur of excess water.

Then dice the cucumber, bell pepper and tomato. Add the bulgur through spring onions to a large bowl and gently stir to distribute ingredients evenly.

In a small separate bowl, whisk together the vinegar, mustard, soy sauce, lemon juice and flax. Dress the salad with the dressing and serve the salad on a bed of greens.

One serving is half of the recipe.

1.49 Asian Bok Choy and Mushroom Salad

Ingredients

1 pound of bok choy

1 ½ cups brown button mushrooms

2 medium carrots

3 cups shelled, frozen edamame

½ purple onion, thinly sliced

1 tbsp ginger, fresh and minced

2 tsp sweet paprika

2 tbsp vegetable stock

2 tbsp white wine vinegar

Directions

Prepare the produce: chop the bok choy into medium, bite-sized pieces; dice the mushrooms into medium cubes.

If possible, use a julienne peeler to form noodles out of the carrots. If you don't have a julienne peeler, you can do this by hand or chop them into different shapes.

Next heat a non-stick fry pan (or electric fry pan) to medium heat. Cook the bok choy, onion, carrots, ginger and paprika with the stock in a fry pan for around 4 minutes. Cover but stir frequently. After 4 minutes the bok choy should be partially cooked and starting to wilt. Add stock by the tablespoon if the mixture is too dry and starts to burn.

Add the mushrooms and vinegar to the pan. Continue to stir the mixture until the mushrooms and bok choy are cooked through, around 4 more minutes.

Enjoy immediately. One serving is half the recipe.

1.50 Middle Eastern Mason jar Salad

Ingredients

1 1/2 tbsp lemon juice

1 1/2 tbsp olive oil

1 tsp Dijon mustard

1 tsp honey

Pinch salt and pepper pinch of each

1/4 cup red bell pepper finely diced

1/4 cup cucumber finely diced

1/2 cup canned chickpeas rinsed and drained

1/4 cup cooked quinoa

1/2 oz feta cheese crumbled

1/3 cup cherry tomatoes sliced in half

2 tbsp olives minced

1 tbsp sunflower seeds

1/2 tsp za'atar

1 cup spinach

Directions

Layer into a 1 L mason jar and enjoy!

1.51 One Pot Cheesy Taco Skillet

Ingredients

1 lb lean ground beef

1 large yellow onion, diced

2 bell peppers, diced

1 12 oz. can diced tomatoes with green chilis

1-2 large zucchinis, diced

2 tbsp taco seasoning

3 cups baby kale/spinach mixture, this sounds like a lot- it cooks down to a small amount, optional

1 1/2 cup shredded cheddar and jack cheese

Green onions, to garnish

Directions

In a large pan, lightly brown ground beef and crumble well. Drain excess fat. Add vegetables, and cook until browned. Add canned tomatoes, taco seasoning, and any water needed for taco seasoning to evenly coat mixture (up to 1 tbsp- the liquid from the tomatoes will help)

Add greens and let fully wilt. Mix well.

Cover with shredded cheese, and let cheese melt - about five minutes (sometimes it helps to cover the pan with a lid to melt the cheese faster.)

When cheese is melted, serve over a bed of lettuce, rice, or in a taco or burrito! Garnish with green onions if desired.

1.52 Lamb Stew with Mushrooms & Red Wine

Ingredients

3 lb lamb leg, cut into 1-inch cubes

4 tbsp. cooking fat of choice, divided (like duck fat and avocado oil)

Sea salt and freshly cracked pepper, to taste

1 med. yellow onion, diced

4 medium carrots, divided

2 c sliced cremini mushrooms

1 c dry red wine, like cabernet

1 tbsp. tomato paste

1 tsp. anchovy paste

1 bay leaf

1/2 tsp. crushed dried rosemary

1/2 tsp. dried marjoram

1/2 tsp. dried thyme

4 c beef bone broth

1 small bulb fennel, diced

1 medium parsnip, peeled and diced

1 large celery root, peeled and diced

2 tbsp. arrowroot powder

2 tbsp. water

Directions

In a large, heavy-bottomed soup pot, melt 2 T. cooking fat over medium-high heat. Add lamb, sprinkle with salt and pepper and brown on all sides. Remove lamb from pot with a slotted spoon, and set aside.

Add onion, 1 carrot (peeled and diced small), and mushrooms to cooking juices in pot. Cook stirring over medium-high heat, 5 to 7 minutes or until softened.

Add wine. Bring to a boil, scraping any browned bits from bottom of pan. Let bubble until wine is reduced by half.

Add tomato paste, anchovy paste, bay leaf, herbs, and broth. Bring to a boil, reduce heat, cover and simmer over medium-low heat, 45 minutes or until meat is tender.

Preheat oven to 450 F. On a large, rimmed baking sheet, toss remaining 3 carrots, fennel, parsnip, and celery root with remaining 2 T. cooking fat (melted if necessary), sea salt and freshly ground pepper, to taste. Place in oven and roast 20-30 minutes or until tender and beginning to brown.

Once lamb is tender, add roasted veggies to stew. In a small cup combine arrowroot powder with 2 T. water, and whisk with a fork until smooth. Add arrowroot slurry to stew and bring to a simmer until broth has thickened. Taste and adjust seasoning with sea salt and freshly ground pepper, and enjoy!

1.53 Lentil Stew

Ingredients

1 lb or 450g brown lentils

4 large carrots, chopped

4 medium celery sticks, chopped

1 bay leaf

2 teaspoon chopped fresh thyme or 4 teaspoons dry thyme

1 large yellow onion

4 tablespoons olive oil

4 cloves garlic, chopped

2 teaspoons cumin seeds, roasted and ground

3 teaspoons sea salt

1 lemon, juice

Freshly ground black pepper

2 cups or 500g chicken stock

1/3 cup cilantro, chopped

1 cup parsley, chopped

Directions

It is recommended that you soak the lentils overnight – this is to remove the physic acid which is often a problem for people with digestive issues. If you are not experiencing digestive issues, rinsing the lentils will do.

Put the lentils in a pot with 10 cups of filtered water, add vegetables and bay leaf.

Bring water to boil and lower the heat to simmer for about 1 hour.

Meantime, sauté the onions in oil until soft, then add garlic and continue sautéing till brow.

Add the onions and garlic to your soup as it simmers.

Add chicken stock, lemon juice, cumin and salt in the last 15 minutes of cooking.

Turn off the heat and add cilantro and parsley.

Correct the seasoning with salt, pepper or cumin.

1.54 Vegetable Soup with Mediterranean Salad

Ingredients

1 can diced tomatoes (no salt added, 14 oz.)

2 oz. frozen spinach

½ lb. frozen green beans

5 oz. frozen or canned corn

1 medium/large carrot, grated

1 tsp dry oregano

1 tsp garlic powder

1 tsp paprika

1 tbsp basil

2 cups water/stock

2 cups lettuce blend

¼ c fresh parsley, finely chopped

2 ripe roma tomatoes, diced

1 tbsp flax seed

2 tbsp red wine vinegar

2-4 tbsp water

Black pepper, to taste

Directions

Add ingredients from the canned tomatoes through basil into a medium saucepan. Cover the ingredients with the liquid. Place the saucepan on high heat, cover with a lid and bring it to a boil. Once boiling, turn down the mixture to allow it to simmer. Simmer the soup for 10 minutes, stirring occasionally.

After 10 minutes, uncover the soup. Allow the soup to cook for 10 minutes. Then turn the heat off and allow the soup to cool while you prepare the salad.

For the salad: add the lettuce blend to a bowl. Top with chopped parsley and diced tomatoes. In a separate bowl, whisk together the flax, vinegar and water. Drizzle the salad with the dressing.

Enjoy the soup and salad together.

1.55 Slow Cooker Vegetarian Chili

Ingredients

2 teaspoons canola oil

1 large onion, diced

2 stalks celery, diced

2 carrots, diced

2 cloves garlic, chopped

1 bell pepper, diced

2 tablespoons dark chili powder

2 teaspoons ground cumin

1/4 teaspoon red pepper flakes

1 (29-ounce) can crushed tomatoes

3 (15.5 oz) cans red kidney or black beans, rinsed and drained

12 ounces butternut squash, peeled and diced (about 3 cups)

1 cup vegetable stock

Directions

Note: Sautéing the vegetables before adding them to the slow cooker creates a layer of flavor. Do not skip this step.

Heat the oil in a saute pan, then add the onions, carrots and celery. Saute for four minutes, until the vegetables start to soften. Add the garlic and bell pepper, stir and saute another 2 minutes.

Add the spices and cook for one minute, stirring constantly. Remove the pan from heat.

Add the vegetables and the remaining ingredients to the slow cooker and stir to combine. Cover and cook on low for six hours.

1.56 Pumpkin Turkey Chili

Ingredients

2 tablespoons avocado oil or ghee

1 yellow onion, chopped

2 cloves garlic, finely chopped

1 red bell pepper, cored, seeded and chopped

1 jalapeño, seeded and finely chopped

1 pound ground turkey (or leftover turkey)

2 tablespoons chili powder

2 teaspoons ground cumin

1 (14.5-ounce) can diced tomatoes, with their liquid

1 (15-ounce) can pumpkin purée

1½ cups water

1 teaspoon sea salt

Ground black pepper, to taste

1 (15-ounce) canned kidney beans, rinsed and drained

Directions

Heat oil or ghee in a large pot over medium high heat. Add onion, garlic, bell pepper, and jalapeño and sauté until they begin to soften, about 4-5 minutes.

Add turkey, cumin, and chili powder. Using a wooden spoon or spatula, break turkey up into smaller bits and cook until meat is browned.

Add tomatoes, pumpkin, water, salt, and pepper and bring to a boil. Reduce heat to medium low and add beans. Cover and simmer, stirring occasionally, for at least 15-20 minutes to allow flavors to meld.

Ladle into bowls and serve.

Note: If you have leftover cooked turkey from Thanksgiving, simply substitute it for the ground turkey. Since it's already been cooked, you can add it to the pot at the same time as the tomatoes, pumpkin, water, and spices.

1.57 Sweet & Spicy Quinoa Chili

Ingredients

3/4 c dry quinoa, sprouted (yields around 1 cup)

1/3 c dry brown lentils, sprouted (yields around 1 cup)

1 c dry black beans, sprouted

1 c dry pinto beans, sprouted

1 can diced tomatoes (no salt added)

1/2 onion, diced

1 red bell pepper, diced

1/4 c fresh cilantro, diced

4 large cloves garlic, minced

1 tbsp blackstrap molasses

1 lime, juiced

1 tbsp cinnamon

1 tbsp paprika

1 tsp chili powder

1/2 tsp ground cloves

1/2 tsp white pepper

1/2 tsp black pepper

1/2 tsp chili flakes

1/4 tsp turmeric

1/4 tsp cumin

2 1/2 c vegetable stock (low/no sodium)

Directions

Add all ingredients into a pressure cooker. Stir well.

Lock the lid and bring to pressure.

Cook at full pressure for 20 minutes.

Quick release when finished. Enjoy.

1.58 Easy Mexican Black Beans with Greens

Ingredients

1 can diced tomatoes (no salt added, 14 oz.)

1 carrot, grated

1 cup black beans soaked in 2 cups water overnight*

½ onion, diced

½ tbsp minced garlic

1 tbsp dry parsley flakes

1 tbsp vinegar (your choice)

2 tsp paprika

2 tsp cumin

1 tsp oregano flakes

½ tsp chili flakes (or to taste)

½ tsp chili powder (or to taste)

¼ tsp black pepper (or to taste)

Salad greens

Directions

Prepare all the ingredients as noted. Add the ingredients to a medium-large pressure cooker. Mix the ingredients and secure the lid.

Pressure cook the mixture for 3 minutes. After 8 minutes, quick release the cooker to remove from pressure.

To enjoy, plate as many salad greens as you want and top with 1-1 ½ cups of your Mexican Black Bean recipe. Feel free to add more veggies to your salad.

1.59 Summer Squash Skillet

Ingredients

1 cup summer squash, sliced

1 cup zucchini, sliced

1/4 cup carrots, strips or slices

5 medium fresh mushrooms

1/2 tbsp ghee

Seasoned salt

Directions

Cut squash, carrots and mushrooms in thin slices.

Melt ghee in skillet; add vegetables and seasoned salt. Cook until slightly browned; turn and cook until underside is browned.

Mushroom Leek Stir Fry

Ingredients

3 cups oyster mushrooms (you can also use shiitake), sliced and roots removed

1 cup sprouted beans

1 onion, sliced thinly

2 leeks, sliced to rings

3 cloves of crushed garlic

1 inch of minced ginger

1 tsp cumin

1 carrot, sliced

5 oz (150g) rice noodles (omit if you are doing GAPS)

½ cup soy (aka tamari) sauce (or coconut aminos if you are off soy)

½ tsp chili

1 tbsp coconut oil

Directions

Boil the rice noodles as per instructions given, set aside in cold water.

Heat coconut oil, throw in cumin for 30 seconds till fragrant.

Add onion, garlic and ginger and fry on high heat for 3 min.

Add leeks and continue frying till slightly browned.

Add mushrooms, sprouted beans and carrot, and stir fry till mushrooms become soft.

Add soy sauce and chili.

Add noodles and let the sauce bring all the ingredients together.

Cook for 2 more minutes, stirring occasionally.

Serve warm.

One of the great things about a stir fry is improvisation. Whatever you have in the fridge, just throw it in and it will blend in deliciously.

1.60 Baked Risotto Primavera

Ingredients

1 tablespoon oil, olive, extra-virgin

2 medium onions chopped, (about 1 1/2 cups)

1 cup rice, brown medium- or short-grain

3 cloves garlic minced

1/2 cup wine, dry white

29 ounces broth, chicken, less sodium or 3 1/2 cups vegetable broth

8 ounces asparagus ends trimmed, cut into 1-inch pieces

1 cup peas, sugar snap or snow peas, trimmed, cut into 1-inch pieces

1 cup peppers, red, bell diced, (about 1 medium)

1 1/2 cups cheese, Parmesan freshly grated 1/4 cup parsley, fresh chopped

1/4 cup chives, fresh chopped

2 teaspoon lemon zest (1 - 2 teaspoons as desired)

Pepper, black ground to taste

Directions

Preheat oven to 425 degrees F.

Heat oil in a Dutch oven or ovenproof high sided skillet over medium heat. Add onions and cook, stirring occasionally, until softened, 3 to 5 minutes.

Stir in rice and garlic; cook, stirring, 1 to 2 minutes. Stir in wine and simmer until it has mostly evaporated. Add broth and bring to a boil. Cover the pan and transfer to the oven.

Bake until the rice is just tender, 50 minutes to 1 hour.

Shortly before the risotto is done, steam asparagus, peas, and bell pepper until crisp-tender, about 4 minutes.

Fold the steamed vegetables, Parmesan, parsley, chives, lemon zest, and pepper into the risotto. Serve immediately.

1.61 Rosemary Roasted Potatoes and Tomatoes

Ingredients

1 pound potatoes, new (tiny) scrubbed and quartered

2 tablespoons oil, olive

1 teaspoon rosemary, snipped

1/4 teaspoon salt

1/4 teaspoon pepper, black, ground

4 tomatoes, plum, quartered lengthwise

1/2 cup olives, Kalamata, pitted, halved

3 cloves garlic, minced

Directions

Preheat oven to 450°F. Lightly grease a 15x10x1-inch baking pan; place potatoes in pan.

In a small bowl, combine oil, rosemary, salt, and pepper; drizzle over potatoes, tossing to coat.

Bake for 20 minutes, stirring once. Add tomatoes, olives, and garlic, tossing to combine. Bake for 5 to 10 minutes more or until potatoes are tender and brown on the edges and tomatoes are soft.

Transfer to a serving dish. Sprinkle with Parmesan cheese.

1.62 Moroccan Bean

Ingredients

1 can of mixed beans, drained (reserve liquid)

1 onion, diced

3 cloves garlic, minced

3 medium tomatoes, finely diced

1/4 cup lemon juice (juice of 1/2 lemon)

2 tsp chili powder

2 dry chilies, minced

1 tsp chili flakes

1 tbsp cumin

2 tsp paprika

1/2 tsp to thyme

1 Tbsp dry parsley

Black pepper, lightly to taste (1/2-1 tsp)

Water or vegetable stock

Brown rice, to serve

Directions

Sauté onions and garlic in a large fry pan for a few minutes until they are cooked through and translucent.

Add the tomatoes and sauté for another few minutes until the tomatoes have softened.

Next add the spices and lemon juice, adding enough liquid (water or vegetable stock) to keep the mixture moist and from sticking to the bottom of the pan. Allow the flavors to blend in the pan for around 5 minutes, adding more liquid as necessary.

Finally add the drained beans and half of the bean liquid to the fry pan. Keep moving the contents of the pan around to ensure that the beans get evenly and thoroughly heated through. The beans are done when they are thoroughly heated.

Serve beans over pre-cooked brown rice and enjoy immediately.

1.63 Saucy Vegan Vegetable & Chickpea Curry

Ingredients

Curry Spice Mix

1 tsp chili powder

1/2 tsp black pepper

2 tsp fenugreek (methi)

1/2 tsp ginger

2 tsp turmeric

1 tsp cumin powder

1/2 tsp mustard powder

1/4 tsp cardamom

1/8 tsp cloves

Chickpea Curry

1 curry spice mix (see above)

1 onion, diced

5 large cloves garlic, diced

2 tbsp white vinegar

215 g (1/2 lb) frozen cauliflower, chopped

2 carrots, diced

1 1/2 c sweet potato leaves, chopped (spinach works, too)

1 can diced tomatoes (salt free)

1 c water

2 c cooked chickpeas

Directions

Heat large fry pan to high heat. Add the onions and garlic the pan. Sauté the onions and garlic, stirring frequently, between 3-5 minutes. The onions should caramelize and turn a light golden brown.

Next add chili powder, black pepper, fenugreek, ginger and a small amount of liquid to the pan. Toast the spices for a few minutes before adding 1/2 cup water. Cook the mixture for a few more minutes.

Add the carrots, cauliflower, tomatoes, leaves, the other 1/2 cup water and the rest of the spices.

Simmer the mixture for 10 minutes.

Serve with whole wheat sourdough roti or wholegrain rice. Enjoy.

1.64 Curried Lamb & Fennel Meatballs in Tomato Sauce

Ingredients

2 tbsp. ghee, divided

1 medium bulb fennel, minced

1 tbsp. curry powder

1 medium shallot, minced

2 cloves garlic, minced

2 lb ground lamb

1 egg

1 tsp. fine sea salt

Freshly ground pepper, to taste

14 1/2 oz can tomato sauce

1 1/2 c whole milk greek-style yogurt, plain

1/3 c pine nuts, toasted*/ toasted sliced almonds

A handful of fresh cilantro leaves

Directions

In a large skillet- over medium-high heat, melt 1 tablespoon ghee. Add fennel and saute until tender, 3 - 5 minutes. Add curry powder, shallot, and garlic and saute one minute more. Remove from heat and set aside until cool enough to handle.

In a medium mixing bowl combine ground lamb, egg, salt, and pepper. Add fennel mixture and mix to combine. Form into walnut-sized balls.

In same large skillet, melt remaining ghee over medium-high heat. Add meatballs and brown, undisturbed, about 5 minutes. Flip once and brown again for another 5 minutes. Add tomato sauce, bring to a simmer and reduce heat. Simmer 15 minutes uncovered, or until meatballs are cooked through and sauce has thickened a bit.

Serve with yogurt, toasted pine nuts, and fresh cilantro.

1.65 Moroccan Chicken

Ingredients

2 pounds chicken, pieces (breast halves, thighs, and drumsticks) skinned finely shredded

1/2 cup orange juice

1 tablespoon oil, olive

1 tablespoon ginger, fresh

1 teaspoon paprika

1 teaspoon cumin, ground

1/2 teaspoon coriander, ground

1/4 teaspoon pepper, red, crushed

1/8 teaspoon salt

2 teaspoons orange peel

2 tablespoons honey

2 teaspoons orange juice

Directions

Place chicken in a large resealable plastic bag set in a deep dish.

For marinade, in a small bowl, stir together the 1/2 cup orange juice, the olive oil, ginger, paprika, cumin, coriander, crushed red pepper, and salt. Pour marinade over chicken. Seal bag; turn to coat chicken.

Marinate in the refrigerator for at least 4 hours or up to 24 hours, turning the bag occasionally.

Meanwhile, in a small bowl, stir together orange peel, honey, and the 2 teaspoons orange juice.

Drain the chicken, discarding the marinade.

Prepare grill for indirect grilling. Test for medium heat above pan. Place chicken, skinned sides up, on lightly greased grill rack over drip pan.

Cover and grill for 50 to 60 minutes or until chicken is done (170°F for breast halves; 180°F for thighs and drumsticks); brush occasionally with honey mixture during the last 10 minutes of grilling.

1.66 Quinoa Crusted Chicken Parmesan

Ingredients

3-4 chicken breasts, sliced in half and pounded to thin cutlets (about 1 1/2 pounds)

1 1/2 cups lactose free milk

1/2 cup potato starch

Salt and pepper, to taste

2 eggs

2 cups cooked quinoa

2 teaspoons chopped basil

1/4 cup Parmesan cheese

1 cup marinara sauce (low FODMAP variety such as Rao's Sensitive Formula)

1 cup shredded mozzarella cheese

Fresh sliced basil for garnish if desired

Directions

Preheat oven to 375 degrees F.

Lightly oil large baking sheet.

In medium bowl, add milk and chicken breasts, set aside.

Place potato starch on plate and sprinkle with salt and pepper, set aside.

In small bowl, add eggs and whisk to blend, set aside.

Place quinoa in bowl and add basil, stir to blend, set aside.

Take one chicken cutlet out of milk and dip lightly on both sides in potato starch, shake to remove excess starch.

Dip starch coated chicken into eggs to coat and then into quinoa.

Press quinoa firmly into chicken breast, then place chicken on baking sheet.

Repeat process with the rest of the chicken.

Sprinkle Parmesan cheese over chicken breasts, evenly.

Bake for 25 minutes or until cooked through. Remove from oven carefully and add 2 tablespoons of marinara over each breast and top with a sprinkle of the mozzarella cheese.

Return to the oven for 5 minutes to melt cheese and heat sauce; top with fresh sliced basil if desired.

1.67 Chicken Cilantro

Ingredients

For the Chicken:

2 chicken breasts, skinless, bone-in halves (cut in two if they're large)

2 chicken thighs, skinless, bone-in

2 chicken drumsticks

2 tbsp. olive oil

1 1/2 bunches cilantro, divided

1 medium white onion, peeled and roughly chopped

6 cloves garlic

14 fl oz chicken broth

Salt and pepper, to taste

For the Rice:

2 c long grain white rice

1/2 c minced onion, preferably white

1 tbsp. butter or ghee

3 sprigs cilantro

1 lime, juice only

3 c water or chicken broth

Salt and pepper, to taste

Directions

For the Chicken:

If you haven't already, remove skin from chicken breasts and thighs-- the drumsticks will hold together better if you leave the skin on. Rinse chicken under cool running water, and pat dry. Sprinkle chicken generously with salt and pepper on both sides.

Heat oil in a large dutch oven with a tight-fitting lid over medium-high heat. Saute until nicely browned, 5-10 minutes each side.

Meanwhile, combine 1 bunch cilantro, onion, garlic, and chicken broth in blender. Once blended, pour over chicken and simmer, covered, until meat is fork-tender and easily pulls away from the bone, about 45 minutes.

Taste and adjust seasoning. Serve over Maria's Rice, garnished with plenty of fresh cilantro leaves.

For the Rice:

In a sauce pan with a tight-fitting lid, melt butter or ghee over medium heat. Add rice and onion, and cook, stirring, until rice becomes opaque, about 2-3 minutes. Add whole cilantro sprigs, lime juice, water or broth, and salt to taste. Bring to a boil, reduce heat, cover and simmer 20 minutes (or according to package instructions). Remove heat and let stand, covered, 10 minutes more. Remove cilantro sprigs, fluff with a fork, and serve.

1.68 Maple-Chili Glazed Pork Medallions

Ingredients

1 teaspoon chili powder

1/2 teaspoon salt

1/8 teaspoon peppers, chipotle chile, ground

1 pound pork, lean tenderloin trimmed and cut crosswise into 1-inch think medallions

2 teaspoons oil, canola

1/4 cup apple cider

1 tablespoon maple syrup

1 teaspoon vinegar, cider

Directions

Mix chili powder, salt, and ground chipotle in a small bowl. Sprinkle over both sides of pork.

Heat oil in a large skillet over medium-high heat. Add the pork and cook until golden, 1 to 2 minutes per side.

Add cider, syrup, and vinegar to the pan. Bring to a boil, scraping up any browned bits.

Reduce the heat to medium and cook, turning the pork occasionally to coat, until the sauce is reduced to a thick glaze, 1 to 3 minutes. Serve the pork drizzled with the glaze.

1.69 Southwestern Steak and Peppers

Ingredients

1/2 tablespoon cumin, ground

1/2 teaspoon coriander, ground

1/2 teaspoon chili powder

1/4 teaspoon salt

3/4 teaspoon pepper, black, coarsely ground

1 pound beef, boneless top sirloin steak trimmed of fat

3 cloves garlic, peeled, 1 halved and 2 minced

3 teaspoons oil, canola divided (or olive oil)

2 medium peppers, red, bell thinly sliced

1 medium onion, white halved lengthwise and thinly sliced

1 teaspoon sugar, brown

1/2 cups coffee, brewed or prepared instant coffee

1/4 cup vinegar, balsamic

4 cups watercress

Directions

Mix cumin, coriander, chili powder, salt, and 3/4 teaspoon pepper in a small bowl. Rub steak with the cut garlic. Rub the spice mix all over the steak.

Heat 2 teaspoons oil in a large heavy skillet, preferably cast iron, over medium-high heat. Add the steak and cook to desired doneness, 4 to 6 minutes per side for medium-rare. Transfer to a cutting board and let rest.

Add remaining 1 teaspoon oil to the skillet. Add bell peppers and onion; cook, stirring often, until softened, about 4 minutes. Add minced garlic and brown sugar; cook, stirring often, for 1 minute. Add coffee, vinegar, and any accumulated meat juices; cook for 3 minutes to intensify flavor. Season with pepper.

To serve, mound 1 cup watercress on each plate. Top with the sautéed peppers and onion. Slice the steak thinly across the grain and arrange on the vegetables. Pour the sauce from the pan over the steak. Serve immediately.

1.70 Smoky Stuffed Peppers

Ingredients

6 large peppers, bell, any color tops cut off, seeded

12 ounces sausage, Italian turkey, hot links, removed from casings

1 1/2 cups broth, chicken, less sodium

4 medium tomatoes, plum chopped

2 cups rice, brown, instant

1 cup basil, fresh chopped

1 cup cheese, smoked mozzarella (or smoked cheddar or Gouda), finely shredded, divided

Directions

Position rack in upper third of oven; preheat broiler.

Place peppers cut-side down in a large microwave-safe dish. Fill the dish with 1/2 inch of water, cover and microwave on High until the peppers are just softened, 7 to 10 minutes. Drain the water and transfer the peppers to a roasting pan.

Meanwhile, cook sausage in a large non-stick skillet over medium-high heat, breaking it up into small pieces with a wooden spoon, until cooked through, about 5 minutes.

Stir in broth, tomatoes, and rice; increase heat to high and bring to a simmer. Cover, reduce heat to medium-low and simmer until the rice is softened but still moist, 5 minutes. Remove from the heat and let stand, covered, until the rice absorbs the remaining liquid, about 5 minutes.

Stir basil and half the cheese into the rice mixture. Divide the filling among the peppers, then top with the remaining cheese. Broil until the cheese is melted, 2 to 3 minutes.

1.71 Steamed Artichokes with Garlic Cashew Aioli

Ingredients:

4 artichokes

1 cup cashews

2 tablespoons olive oil

3 garlic cloves

2 lemons

¼ teaspoon sea salt

½ to 1 cup water

Directions

Trim the artichokes by slicing ½ inch off of the tops and all but ½ inch off the stems. Trim any remaining leaves by ½ inch as well. Bring a pot of water to boil. Place the artichokes into a steamer basket inside the pot. Steam the artichokes for 30 to 40 minutes depending on size. They're done when one of the leaves pulls off easily and is tender.

Combine the cashews, olive oil, and garlic, juice of two lemons, and sea salt in the blender with ½ cup of water. Blend until smooth for a thicker aioli. For a thinner consistency, continue to stream in another ½ cup of water while blending.

Serve the artichokes alongside the cashew aioli for dipping and top with any fresh herbs as desired!

1.72 Sweet Italian Sausage

Ingredients

3 tbsp. EVOO

2 c finely diced onion, about 1 1/2 medium (or sub. 1 T onion powder)

1 1/2 tbsp. Italian Herb Seasoning

1 1/2 tsp. ground fennel

3/4 tsp. paprika

3/4 tsp. red chili flakes (for mild heat)

1 tbsp. honey

1/4 c plus 2 tbsp. freshly minced garlic, about 6-8 cloves (or sub. 1 T. garlic powder)

3 lb ground pork

1 tbsp. fine sea salt

3/4 tsp. freshly ground black pepper

3 tbsp. red wine vinegar

Directions

In a medium skillet, over medium heat, combine olive oil and onion. Cook 3-5 minutes or until soft (no color).

While onions are cooking add Italian herbs, ground fennel, paprika, chili flakes, and honey. NOTE: If using onion powder, simply add with other herbs and spices to the oil, and heat to help the flavors 'bloom', until fragrant, 1 - 2 minutes.

Add chopped garlic to the pan and cook 1 minute more or until fragrant (no color). Remove pan from heat and let cool for a couple minutes.

In a medium mixing bowl combine ground pork, sea salt, black pepper, and red wine vinegar. Use a heat-proof rubber spatula to scrape in the herb and spice oil. Mix with your hands to combine. Use or freeze as desired.

1.73 Loaded Lasagna

Ingredients

Cheesy Sauce:

2 cups chickpeas, sprouted

2 tbsp lemon juice

1/2 tsp black pepper

1/2 cup sauerkraut

1 tbsp ground mustard

Marinara Sauce:

3 cloves garlic, minced

1 brown onion, diced

1/4 cup red wine (vinegar if unavailable)

2 tsp oregano

2 tbsp dry parsley

2 tsp dry thyme

1 lb (500-600 grams) fresh tomatoes, diced (or 1 can)

Noodles:

1 lb (600 g) zucchini, sliced lengthwise

Chopped Veggie Ideas (at least 2 are recommended):

Carrots

Mushrooms

Capsicum

Spinach

Directions

Marinara Sauce:

Sauté the onions and garlic in a fry pan with half the wine for 5 minutes or until the onions are slightly translucent. Add the oregano, parsley and thyme and cook for a few more minutes.

Lastly add the tomatoes and the rest of the wine. Occasionally stir the contents of the pan until the tomatoes have broken down and juices have come out. Simmer for 15 minutes or until a thick sauce has formed. Set aside.

Cheesy Sauce:

Slightly overcook the chickpeas (pressure cook for 18 minutes or on stovetop for necessary time). Add the chickpeas, lemon juice, black pepper, sauerkraut and mustard into your blender or food processor. Blend the ingredients into a smooth sauce. If you need to add extra water to the mixture in order to blend it, use excess water leftover from cooking the chickpeas. Use as little water as possible in order to purée. Set aside.

Noodles:

Slice off both ends of the zucchini. Using a mandolin or another slicer of the sort, slice the zucchini lengthwise into long, thin and wide strips. Do this for all the zucchini. Set aside.

Vegetables:

Chop, slice, grate or dice your selected filling vegetables as desired and set aside.

Assembly and Baking:

Preheat oven to 350° F (180° C).

Lay the zucchini noodles along the bottom of a large oven-save baking dish.

First cover the zucchini in a layer of cheese sauce, then the tomato sauce and lastly sprinkle chopped vegetables on top. Repeat the process of covering the dish with noodles, sauce and chopped veggies.

End with a layer of zucchini on the top. Bake covered for 20 minutes, uncover and bake for another 15 minutes.

Remove from oven and enjoy after allowing the lasagna to cool for 5-10 minutes as the contents of the dish will be extremely hot.

1.74 Stuffed Delicata Squash with Sausage, Greens, & Garlic

Ingredients

4 medium delicata squash

A knob of ghee or other cooking fat

1 medium yellow onion, diced small

2 tbsp. minced garlic

1 lb sweet Italian sausage (pork or turkey)

1 1/2 tsp. rubbed sage

1/8 tsp. grated nutmeg

Pinch red chili flakes, or more to taste

1/2 tsp. fine sea salt, or more to taste

Few grinds black pepper

6 c roughly chopped chard leaves (stems removed)

2/3 c finely grated Parmesan cheese

2/3 c finely grated Romano cheese

1/3 c pine nuts, toasted (optional but recommended)

Directions

Preheat oven to 350. Wash the squash and cut lengthwise, through the middle. Use a spoon to scrape the seeds and stringy flesh from the squash halves. Place the squash halves cut side down onto a parchment-lined baking sheet and place in oven, 25 to 30 minutes or until the squash gives a little when squeezed.

While squash are baking, heat ghee in a large, high-sided skillet over medium-high heat. Choose a pot big and deep enough to accommodate the greens. Add diced onion and sauté 3 minutes or until softened.

Add minced garlic and sauté another 2 minutes.

Add sausage, herbs, and seasonings and cook, stirring until meat has browned. Add greens to the pot and stir until they begin to wilt. You may need to add about ¼ cup water or broth to the pot (for steam) if the mixture is too dry, but the meat and greens should release some liquid as they cook. Reduce heat to medium low, cover pot, and cook until greens are tender, stirring occasionally. Taste for doneness. Remove from heat and stir in half of parmesan and Romano cheeses. Taste filling and adjust seasonings. It should be pretty robust, so add salt to taste if necessary.

When squash is tender, remove from oven and arrange cut side up on baking sheet (you can use the same parchment-lined one). Divide the filling evenly among the halves. Top with remaining cheese.

Return to oven for 20 to 30 minutes or until cheese is melted and everything is heated through (this will take longer if they've been refrigerated overnight). Top with toasted pine nuts or toasted, sliced almonds and enjoy!

1.75 Healthy Chipotle Chicken Sweet Potato Skins

Ingredients

3 medium sweet potatoes

3/4 pound boneless skinless chicken breast about 2 small

1/4 cups olive oil

2 tablespoon fresh lime juice

2 cloves garlic minced or grated

3 whole chipotle pepper minced

1 teaspoon dried oregano

1 teaspoon cumin

2 teaspoons chili powder

Salt and pepper

2 cups spinach half a 10oz bag

5 ounces sharp white cheddar cheese grated

Chopped cilantro for garnish

Greek yogurt for serving

Directions

Preheat your oven to 350 degrees.

Wash your sweet potatoes and prick all over with a fork. Place in the oven and bake for 50-60 minutes or until fork tender. Place your chicken in a baking dish and rub with a tablespoon of olive oil, salt and pepper.

Place in the oven with the potatoes and bake for 25 minutes. Allow to cool and shred the chicken with a fork or your hands. When the sweet potatoes are done cut in half and allow to cool for 5-10 minutes.

In a medium size bowl combine the olive oil, lime juice, garlic, chipotle peppers, oregano, cumin, chili powder, salt and pepper. Set aside.

Heat a small skillet over medium heat and wilt the spinach (this can also be done in the microwave). Toss the spinach and shredded chicken together, set aside and keep warm.

Turn the oven up to 400 degrees. Scrape the sweet potato out of the peel, leaving a medium size layer of flesh inside with the peel so that it can stand up on its own and place in a baking dish. Brush the skins with a little of the chipotle sauce and bake for 5-10 minutes until nice and crisp.

While the skins bake mix the spinach, chicken and chipotle sauce together. Remove skins from the oven and stuff with the chicken mixture, top with shredded cheese and bake for 10 minutes or until the cheese has melted and the skins are hot and crisp.

Serve with fresh chopped cilantro and Greek yogurt if desired.

1.76 Loaded Chili

Ingredients

A knob of ghee

1 green bell pepper, diced small

1 small onion, diced small

1 tbsp. minced garlic

1 tsp. Lawry's Seasoned Salt, or more to taste

1 tbsp. chili powder

1/2 tsp. chipotle powder, or cayenne, or more to taste

1 tsp. ground cumin

1/2 tsp. ground oregano

1 lb lean ground bison, beef, or turkey

2 (4 oz.) cans diced green chilies

1 (14.5 oz.) can black beans, drained and rinsed

1 (14.5 oz.) can organic fire roasted tomatoes with green chilies, or substitute plain diced tomatoes

1 (8 oz.) can tomato sauce

2/3 c frozen corn kernels

2 tbsp. creamy peanut butter

2 c beef broth, preferably homemade

Salt and pepper, to taste

1 lb sweet potato, peeled and cut into 1/2' dice

A knob of coconut oil

Salt and pepper, to taste

1 fresh lime, cut into wedges

1 c sour cream

1 1/2 c grated cheddar cheese

1 avocado, diced

Directions

In a large soup pot, melt ghee over medium-high heat. Add bell pepper and onion and saute until soft and translucent, 3 - 5 minutes.

Add minced garlic and saute 1 minute more.

Season with Lawry's, chili powder, chipotle powder, cumin, and oregano. Stir to combine and cook 1 minute more.

Add ground meat to pan, and saute until browned, breaking up any large pieces, 3 - 5 minutes.

Add diced green chilies, black beans, diced tomatoes, tomato sauce, corn kernels, peanut butter, and 2 cups beef broth. Stir to combine.

Bring to a boil, reduce heat and let simmer 1 hour to allow flavors to combine. If necessary, add remaining beef broth to thin it.

While chili simmers, preheat oven to 350. Peel sweet potato and chop into 1/2-inch dice.

Place knob of coconut oil on a large, rimmed sheet pan and place in oven until fat is melted. Add sweet potato, sprinkle with salt and pepper, toss with a spatula to coat, and place in center of oven for 20 - 25 mins. or until sweet potato is tender when pierced with a fork.

For garnish: chop lime wedges, grate cheese, and dice avocado. Place in serving dishes and serve alongside hot chili, with sour cream and any other desired toppings (see note below).

1.77 Baked Salmon

Ingredients

4 pieces of salmon

1/4 cup olive oil

1/4 cup lemon juice

4 slices of orange

1 teaspoon of sea salt

Directions

Marinate the salmon in olive oil and lemon juice. Put orange on top of each filet, and sprinkle with sea salt. Bake at 350 F for 30 minutes

1.78 Salmon, Sweet Potato & Watercress Salad with Turmeric Cream

Ingredients

Salmon, Sweet Potato & Watercress Salad

2lb white sweet potatoes, peeled

1 1/2tsp raw apple cider vinegar

1large shallot, peeled and finely chopped

Large handful watercress, roughly chopped

2tbsp capers, roughly chopped

1lb fillet wild sockeye salmon

Lemon wedges to serve

Turmeric Cream

3/4cup coconut cream*

1/4cup olive oil

1/4tsp turmeric

Pinch sea salt

Directions

Cut the sweet potatoes into large chunks and steam for approximately 10 minutes until tender, but not falling apart. Note: the exact cooking time will depend on the size of your chunks. Alternatively, cook them in a large pan of gently simmering water. Once cooked, drain them, pour the vinegar over, and set aside to cool.

Meanwhile, put the dressing ingredients into a bowl and whisk to incorporate. Place it in the refrigerator until needed.

Put the salmon onto a rimmed baking tray and broil, skin side up, for 4-5 minutes or until just cooked. Remove the skin and set aside to cool slightly.

Put the potatoes into a serving bowl, together with the remaining salad ingredients. Give the dressing a good stir and pour over the salad. Combine well. Serve with the lemon wedges.

*Put a can of coconut milk in the refrigerator at least the night before you want to make the recipe.

1.79 Sizzled Citrus Shrimp

Ingredients

3 tablespoons lemon juice

3 tablespoons wine, dry white

2 teaspoons oil, olive, extra-virgin

3 cloves garlic minced

1 pound shrimp, peeled and deveined medium (30-40 per pound)

1 teaspoon oil, olive, extra-virgin

1 whole bay leaf

1/4 teaspoon pepper, red, crushed or 1 dried red chile, halved

1/4 teaspoon salt or to taste

2 tablespoons parsley, fresh chopped

Directions

Combine lemon juice, wine, 2 teaspoons oil, and garlic in a medium bowl. Add shrimp and toss to coat. Cover and marinate in the refrigerator for 15 minutes, tossing occasionally. Drain well, reserving marinade.

Heat 1 teaspoon oil in a large non-stick skillet over medium-high heat. Add shrimp and cook, turning once, until barely pink, about 30 seconds per side; transfer to a plate.

Add bay leaf, crushed red pepper, and the reserved marinade to the pan; simmer for 4 minutes. Return the shrimp and any accumulated juices to the pan; heat through. Season with salt, sprinkle with parsley, and serve immediately.

1.80 Shrimp, Zucchini & Pesto Angel Hair Pasta

Ingredients

1/2 lb shrimp, peeled

4 ounces angel hair, cooking according to package-gluten free, whole wheat

1 zucchini, chopped

1 bell pepper, chopped

1/3 cup prepared or homemade pesto sauce

2 tbsp olive oil

Directions

Prepare pasta according to package.

Add 1 tbsp olive oil to medium high skillet and cook shrimp until brown. Don't stir too much or you won't get a crust! Remove from pan.

Cook pepper and zucchini in remaining olive oil until tender

Toss all together in a bowl with pesto. Serve in bowls.

1.81 Roasted Cod, Tomatoes, Orange, & Onions

Ingredients

1 pound tomatoes, plum firm and small, cut into 1/2-inch-thick wedges

2 medium onions, yellow cut into 1/4-inch-thick wedges

1 tablespoon orange peel (zest), grated finely slivered

1 tablespoon oil, olive, extra-virgin

1 tablespoon thyme leaves chopped

1/2 teaspoon salt, Kosher divided

Pepper, black ground to taste

1 pound fish, cod or other thick-cut, firm-fleshed fish, boneless, skinless, cut into 4 equal portions

4 sprigs thyme, fresh for garnish

Directions

Preheat oven to 400°F.

Combine tomatoes, onions, orange zest, oil, and chopped thyme in a 3-quart glass or ceramic baking dish. Sprinkle with 1/4 teaspoon salt and pepper; stir to combine.

Roast, stirring occasionally, until the onions are golden and brown on the edges, about 45 minutes. Remove from the oven. Increase oven temperature to 450°F.

Push the vegetables aside, add fish and season with the remaining 1/4 teaspoon salt and pepper; spoon the vegetables over the fish.

Return the baking dish to the oven and bake until the fish is opaque in the center, about 10 to 12 minutes. To serve, divide the fish and vegetables among 4 plates and garnish with thyme sprigs.

1.82 Grilled Rosemary-Salmon Skewers

Ingredients

2 teaspoons rosemary, fresh minced

2 teaspoons extra-virgin olive oil

2 cloves garlic minced

1 teaspoon lemon zest freshly grated

1 teaspoon lemon juice

1/2 teaspoon salt, Kosher

1/4 teaspoon pepper, black ground

1 pound fish, salmon fillet center-cut, skinned, cut into 1-inch cubes

1 pint tomatoes, cherry

Directions

Preheat grill to medium-high.

Combine rosemary, oil, garlic, lemon zest, lemon juice, salt, and pepper in a medium bowl. Add salmon; toss to coat. Alternating the salmon and tomatoes, divide among eight 12-inch skewers.

Oil the grill rack. Grill the skewers, carefully turning once, until the salmon is cooked through, 4 to 6 minutes total. Serve immediately.

1.83 Arugula Lemon Pesto

Ingredients

6 oz arugula, washed and dried

1 1/2 tsp. lemon zest

2 large garlic cloves, roughly chopped

3 tbsp. toasted pine nuts, or chopped walnuts

1 tsp. coarse flake sea salt, like Maldon

Few grinds black pepper

1/4 c to 1/3 cup extra virgin olive oil

1 tbsp. plus 1 tsp. lemon juice (or sub. white wine vinegar)

Directions

Combine all ingredients in a food processor and process until very finely minced.

BONUS CHAPTER

Ways to Boost Your Energy with Hypothyroidism

If you have hypothyroidism and you feel like you're dragging yourself through your daily routines, you probably are.

Your thyroid is a small endocrine gland in the front of your neck below your larynx that produces hormones that regulate your metabolism. When it's not producing enough of the hormones called T3 and T4, your body has trouble creating energy from the food that you eat. As a result, your metabolism slows way down. You start to feel tired, sluggish, and maybe even forgetful. On top of that, you start to gain weight.

In other words, you need an energy boost. Try these seven strategies to feel more energized:

Choose cardio.

Aerobic exercise is good for you, regardless of your hypothyroidism. It helps you burn calories to lose any extra pounds you might have gained. Cardiovascular exercise also produces endorphins that will improve your mood. So, get up, get those arms and legs moving, and get your heart rate up. Aim for 150 minutes of moderately intense activity per week.

Lift weights.

Build and maintain muscle mass by incorporating some strength-training exercise into your life. If you're already logging 150 minutes of moderately intense cardiovascular exercise, then the Centers for Disease Control and Prevention suggests adding two weekly strength-training workouts to your calendar. Work on all your major muscle groups for maximum benefit.

Make sure your medication dose is correct.

Doctors typically prescribe a hormone replacement called levothyroxine for people with hypothyroidism it replaces the amount of T4 that your thyroid can't produce. According to the American Thyroid Association, your symptoms should lessen and maybe even disappear if you're taking the correct dose of medicine. However, the appropriate dose may need to change over your lifetime. Additionally, some people find themselves tossing and turning from insomnia at night, and it's possible that their thyroid medication may be a contributing factor. Consult your doctor if you feel like the medicine might not be working as well as it should.

Improve your diet.

If you're dragging yourself to the coffee pot several times a day in search of a caffeine-packed energy boost, consider your diet. Eating a diet that's heavy on the fruits, veggies, whole grains, and lean sources of protein is your goal. Replace full-fat dairy with reduced-fat versions, and consider having a snack of nuts or legumes, which provide protein and micronutrients.

Drink more water.

Speaking of coffee consumption, how much water are you drinking in a typical day? Women should aim for about nine cups of water per day, and men should try to guzzle down about 13 cups. Those are only guidelines, however, and you may need to increase your water consumption if you're exercising, or if the weather is particularly warm.

Take a nap.

You're beat. Try taking a power nap to recoup a little bit of lost energy. The key to a successful nap is length. The National Sleep Foundation recommends taking a 20-minute power nap to ward off that feeling of exhaustion but don't sleep longer than that because you're more likely to feel groggy afterward.

Get moving.

You don't have to plan a full-fledged workout. Even a short walk can make you feel a little more alive and kicking. If you're at work, trying pacing around your office while you're on the phone. Or take a short break and go outside for some fresh air and a brisk walk. Take the stairs instead of the elevator whenever possible. It might also help you warm up, since people with hypothyroidism tend to experience some cold intolerance as a result of their slowed-down metabolism.

Weight Gain and Hypothyroidism

Hypothyroidism is strongly associated with weight gain. In fact, weight gain is one of the most common symptoms of hypothyroidism and is what ultimately leads many people to the diagnosis of thyroid disease.

Managing your weight can be a challenge with an underactive thyroid, which may be caused by Hashimoto's thyroiditis, medication side effects, a goiter, thyroid cancer, removal the thyroid gland, treatment of hyperthyroidism, iodine deficiency (though less likely in the United States), or a number of other conditions.

The Thyroid/Weight Gain Connection

Hypothyroidism has long been associated with weight gain (and hyperthyroidism with weight loss), but the exact biochemical cause of this link is not completely clear. That said, there are several mechanisms that may explain the connection in cases of low thyroid function.

The two most active thyroid hormones, thyroxine (T4) and triiodothyronine (T3), circulate in the body, and they affect your metabolism through their interaction with your:

- Fat cells
- Muscle
- Liver
- Pancreas
- Hypothalamus

Thyroid hormones normally help the body break down fat, and they help the liver and pancreas function to metabolize stored calories to be used for energy. These hormones also help the muscles throughout the body as they use energy. And when there is an adequate amount of thyroid hormones circulating in the body, the hypothalamus, which is a regulator of thyroid hormone in the brain, decreases the amount of thyrotropin regulating hormone (TRH) secretion.

All of these actions can be disrupted when you have decreased thyroid hormones or diminished thyroid function. Along with symptoms of low energy, the body also holds on to calories, storing them as fat, which is especially difficult to burn off and metabolize.

Treatment with thyroid replacement medications does not necessarily induce weight loss, even when optimal thyroid hormone levels are measured on blood tests.

Losing Weight With Hypothyroidism

If you have hypothyroidism, losing weight can be very challenging. Many people think that once you start taking thyroid hormone replacement medications, the weight just falls off. While treatment can help you lose some of the weight you have gained, it takes planning, hard work, diet, exercise, and getting enough sleep to shed a number of pounds.

Determining how far off you are from your ideal weight and body fat can help you assess how much weight you need to lose. A body mass index (BMI) calculator can help you get started.

Another step to weight loss is determining your own basal metabolic rate (BMR), which can help you gauge your metabolism and guide you in coming up with a target calorie intake per day.

Diet

An optimal diet minimizes simple carbohydrates and sugars and focuses on lean proteins and vegetables. A meal plan for hypothyroidism can keep you on track in terms of calorie goals.

If you are struggling to lose weight, consider working with a nutritionist to find a dietary plan that works best for you.

Exercise

Exercise can also help you lose weight. Current guidelines from the Centers for Disease Control and Prevention (CDC) recommend that adults get 150 minutes of moderate exercise and two sessions of muscle-building each week.

However, people with hypothyroidism may need to go beyond these recommendations to lose weight.

Sleep

Sleep deprivation is strongly linked to weight gain, and that association is clear whether you have thyroid disease or not. Getting enough restorative sleep on a regular basis can help prevent weight gain and help you keep weight off.

Conclusion

Hypothyroidism, or an underactive thyroid, is a health condition that affects many people worldwide.

It can cause symptoms like tiredness, weight gain, constipation, low mood, and cold intolerance among many others.

There's no "best" diet, but eating the right nutrients and taking medications can help manage hypothyroidism symptoms, improve thyroid function, and promote overall well-being.

Everyone has different diet needs, but people with hypothyroidism can benefit from a diet rich in whole, nutrient-dense foods like vegetables, fruits, nuts, and fish.

Hypothyroidism, or an underactive thyroid, is a health condition that affects many people worldwide.

It can cause symptoms like tiredness, weight gain, constipation, low mood, and cold intolerance among many others.

There's no "best" diet, but eating the right nutrients and taking medications can help manage hypothyroidism symptoms, improve thyroid function, and promote overall well-being.

Everyone has different diet needs, but people with hypothyroidism can benefit from a diet rich in whole, nutrient-dense foods like vegetables, fruits, nuts, and fish.

Made in the USA
Middletown, DE
20 July 2025